AF333765

FIBROMYALGIA

RISK FACTORS, SYMPTOMS AND TREATMENT

Pain and its Origins, Diagnosis and Treatments

Additional books in this series can be found on Nova's website
under the Series tab.

Additional E-books in this series can be found on Nova's website
under the E-book tab.

Pain Management - Research and Technology

Additional books in this series can be found on Nova's website
under the Series tab.

Additional E-books in this series can be found on Nova's website
under the E-book tab.

FIBROMYALGIA

RISK FACTORS, SYMPTOMS AND TREATMENT

ANTONIO G. TRISTANO

EDITOR

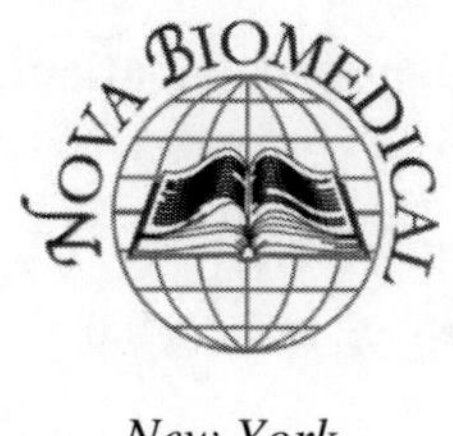

Nova Biomedical

New York

Copyright © 2013 by Nova Science Publishers, Inc.

All rights reserved. No part of this book may be reproduced, stored in a retrieval system or transmitted in any form or by any means: electronic, electrostatic, magnetic, tape, mechanical photocopying, recording or otherwise without the written permission of the Publisher.

For permission to use material from this book please contact us:
Telephone 631-231-7269; Fax 631-231-8175
Web Site: http://www.novapublishers.com

NOTICE TO THE READER

The Publisher has taken reasonable care in the preparation of this book, but makes no expressed or implied warranty of any kind and assumes no responsibility for any errors or omissions. No liability is assumed for incidental or consequential damages in connection with or arising out of information contained in this book. The Publisher shall not be liable for any special, consequential, or exemplary damages resulting, in whole or in part, from the readers' use of, or reliance upon, this material. Any parts of this book based on government reports are so indicated and copyright is claimed for those parts to the extent applicable to compilations of such works.

Independent verification should be sought for any data, advice or recommendations contained in this book. In addition, no responsibility is assumed by the publisher for any injury and/or damage to persons or property arising from any methods, products, instructions, ideas or otherwise contained in this publication.

This publication is designed to provide accurate and authoritative information with regard to the subject matter covered herein. It is sold with the clear understanding that the Publisher is not engaged in rendering legal or any other professional services. If legal or any other expert assistance is required, the services of a competent person should be sought. FROM A DECLARATION OF PARTICIPANTS JOINTLY ADOPTED BY A COMMITTEE OF THE AMERICAN BAR ASSOCIATION AND A COMMITTEE OF PUBLISHERS.

Additional color graphics may be available in the e-book version of this book.

Library of Congress Cataloging-in-Publication Data

ISBN: 978-1-62257-678-4

Library of Congress Control Number: 2012944802

Published by Nova Science Publishers, Inc. † New York

CONTENTS

PREFACE

Fibromyalgia (FM) is a very common disorder, with a prevalence of 2–4% of the population, and about 85–90% of the patients are women. It is defined as a painful syndrome of nonarticular origin characterized by fatigue, widespread musculoskeletal pain, tiredness, and sleep disturbances without any other objective signs or abnormality on examination. Despite being the second commonest syndrome seen often in rheumatology clinics, treatment of FM is frequently unsatisfactory. Many patients also have significant problems in their sexual activity with a chronic or remitting course. Additionally some patients have problems in their oral cavity. Furthermore there is mounting data supporting comorbidity of fibromyalgia syndrome with psychiatric symptoms such as unrefreshing sleep, memory and attention impairment, and syndromes like depression, panic disorder, and post-traumatic stress disorder; these conditions are extremely prevalent ranging from 20 to 80% in clinical samples of patients with FM. The pharmacological management includes several drugs, depending the individual manifestation of this disease, such as: benzodiazepines, non steroidal anti-inflammatory drugs (NSAIDs), analgesics (non-opioid and opioid), anticonvulsivants, serotonin reuptake inhibitors, tricyclic antidepressants, among other. As the concomitance of depression is significantly prevalent in patients affected by fibromyalgia, the use of antidepressant became common in their treatment. However, pathophysiological mechanisms of FM are difficult to identify and current drug therapies demonstrate limited effectiveness, only focused to the management of single symptoms. In general, about half of all treated patients seem to experience a 30% reduction of symptoms, suggesting that many patients with FM will require additional therapies. This book will focus in some aspects not frequently addressed in patients with FM including sexual dysfunction, some comorbidities as oral cavity problems and psychiatric disorders and treatment, principally with antidepressants and complementary medications.

In: Fibromyalgia
Editor: Antonio G. Tristano

ISBN: 978-1-62257-678-4
© 2013 Nova Science Publishers, Inc.

Chapter 1

SEXUAL FUNCTION IN PATIENTS WITH FIBROMYALGIA

Antonio G. Tristano[*]
Rheumatology Department
Centro Médico Docente La Trinidad, Caracas, Venezuela
Centro Médico Carpetana, Madrid, Spain

ABSTRACT

Fibromyalgia is a very common disorder, with a prevalence of 2–12% of the population, and about 85–90% of the patients are women. It is defined as a painful syndrome of nonarticular origin characterized by fatigue, widespread musculoskeletal pain, tiredness, and sleep disturbances without any other objective signs or abnormality on examination. Despite being the second-most-common syndrome seen in rheumatology clinics, treatment of fibromyalgia is frequently unsatisfactory, and many patients have significant problems in their sexual activity with a chronic or remitting course. People with fibromyalgia have a high prevalence of sexual dysfunction, however, only a few studies about sexual function in patients with fibromyalgia have been reported.

There are not enough studies comparing sexual functioning between patients with fibromyalgia and healthy controls. However, there is a

---

[*] E-mail: antoniotristano@yahoo.com. Correspondence address: 5150 NW 99th Ave. Miami, FL, US.

tendency to find more problems with sexual function in patients with fibromyalgia. Sexual dysfunction in patients with fibromyalgia could be principally associated with depression and manifested with diminished desire. However, the characteristic symptoms of fibromyalgia, such as generalized pain, stiffness, fatigue, and poor sleep, may also contribute to the occurrence of sexual dysfunction. This chapter is about the impact of fibromyalgia on sexual functioning.

Keywords: Sexuality; sexual functioning; sexual dysfunction; fibromyalgia

INTRODUCTION

Sexuality has been described as an essential part of the whole person, an integral part of being human, including one's total sense of self, and is linked to the quality of life of the individual. Sexuality is a complex aspect of human life, comprising much more than the act of sexual intercourse. Normal sexual functioning consists of sexual activity with transition through the phases from arousal to relaxation (the desire (appetite), excitement, plateau, orgasm, and resolution phases) with no problems and with a feeling of pleasure, fulfillment and satisfaction [1,2]. Sexual expression has been cited as a crucial part of an individual's self identity and, therefore, is important in all stages of health and illness [3]. Epidemiologic studies in the United States have reported that 30% to 50% of American women complain of sexual dysfunction [4]. Female sexual dysfunction has been classified into four types: hypoactive sexual desire, sexual aversion, and orgasmic and sexual pain disorders. Additionally, sexual pain disorders have been divided into dyspareunia, vaginismus, and anatomic or inflammatory pain disorders. The most common sexual problems in women, accounting for about 20% of the cases, are impaired lubrication and hypoactive sexual activity, arising from the perception of sex as an unpleasant activity [5-8].

On the other hand, rheumatic diseases, including fibromyalgia, may affect all aspects of life including sexual functioning [9]. The reasons for the disturbance of sexual functioning are multifactorial and comprise disease-related factors as well as therapy. These factors include pain, fatigue, stiffness, functional impairment, depression, anxiety, negative body image, reduced libido, hormonal imbalance, and drug treatment [10]. Physical problems, emotional problems and partnership difficulties arising from disease-related stress contribute to a less active and often less enjoyable sex life. Chronic pain, fatigue and low self-esteem can reduce an individual's sexual interest and thereby reduce the frequency of intercourse. The pleasure of intercourse can become diminished by the pain of joint movement or difficulty in finding positions that do not cause discomfort [10].

Sexual problems created by both the physical changes of the illness and its attendant emotional distress not only affect to people with fibromyalgia, but also their partners. Therefore, it is important to consider the marital relationship, and the impact of fibromyalgia on the spouses.

On the other hand, sexual functioning is a neglected area of the quality of life in patients with fibromyalgia and is not routinely addressed by physicians or health professionals, nor is it part of questionnaires frequently used to assess physical function or quality of life. In a recent survey of ten rheumatologists, only 12% of patients seen in their practice were screened for sexual activity. The reasons given by rheumatologists were time constraints, discomfort with the subject, and ambivalence about whether such a screening is in their domain [11].

It is therefore imperative that physicians and nurses raise the subject of sexuality with their patients and it has been suggested that all practicing nurses should reflect on whether they are addressing this topic adequately [12,13].

SEXUAL FUCTION IN PATIENTS WITH FIBROMYALGIA

Fibromyalgia is a very common disorder, with a prevalence of 2% to 12% of the population. Its prevalence increases with age, most dramatically in women with a peak in the fifth to seventh decade (7.4% to 10%). Adult women are affected four to five times more often than adult men [14].

The most common and characteristic symptoms of fibromyalgia are generalized pain, stiffness, fatigue, and poor sleep. However, patients with fibromyalgia may also report a sensation of swelling in the soft tissues and paresthesias. The onset of fibromyalgia symptoms often follows an infection or trauma, as well as mental stress. Depression and mood disorders may also play an important role in the occurrence of fibromyalgia [15,16].

The prevalence of sexual difficulties in patients with chronic pain is high, however, only a few studies about sexual function in patients with fibromyalgia have been reported [17]. Interviews reveal a considerable decrease in the sexual desire of women with fibromyalgia. Questionnaires indicated that fibromyalgia had adversely affected the sex lives of 71% of the patients and that symptoms associated with fibromyalgia affected ability "to make love" in 78% of women [18,19].

Orgasmic problems have been found to be significantly more common in patients with fibromyalgia than in healthy controls, as shown by De Costa et al [20], but they reported no difference in sexual scores between patients and controls. However, this study had significant methodological problems: The sample size was small, the age of the women in fibromyalgia group was significantly higher than that of the controls, and the sexual experience questionnaire was not validated.

After that, Tikiz et al. [21] studied 40 female subjects with fibromyalgia, 27 with fibromyalgia plus major depression and 33 healthy volunteers as a control group. The diagnosis of major depression was made according to Structured Clinical Interview for Diagnostic and Statistical Manual-IV interview, and the Hamilton Depression Rate Scale was used to grade depression. Widespread pain and quality of life were assessed with the Lattinen Pain Scale and Fibromyalgia Impact Questionnaire, respectively. The Female Sexual Function Index (FSFI) was used to assess sexual dysfunction.

They found that the mean FSFI total score was significantly decreased in the fibromyalgia and fibromyalgia plus major depression groups compared with that in healthy controls. However, the FSFI score was not significantly different between patients with fibromyalgia only and fibromyalgia plus major depression. Correlation analysis revealed a negative moderate correlation between total Lattinen pain score and FSFI score in the fibromyalgia only, and fibromyalgia plus major depression group's score did not correlate with FIQ and HDRS scores. They concluded that female patients with fibromyalgia have distinct sexual dysfunction compared with healthy controls, and coexistent major depression has no additional negative effect on sexual function.

In accordance with that, Aydin et al. [22] found similar results. According to the FSFI data, female sexual dysfunction was found in 26 patients with fibromyalgia and only 6 controls, a significant difference. When the subscores of each domain of FSFI were evaluated, the most common sexual problem was diminished desire in patients and controls. They concluded that, particularly, sexual desire and arousal problems appear to be common in premenopausal female patients with fibromyalgia. They also observed that complaints of pain during sexual intercourse were more common in patients with fibromyalgia (50%) than in healthy controls (16.7%).

On the psychiatric evaluation, a depressive mood was more evident and the FSFI score correlated with the STAI and BDI scores in patients with fibromyalgia. Therefore, fibromyalgia, sexual dysfunction, and depression/anxiety may be interrelated, with the depressive mood and anxiety responsible for desire and arousal problems in those patients.

Later, Shaver et al. [23] performed a telephone survey of 442 women with and 205 women without fibromyalgia to assess their health status; data were compared on general health status, reproductive and sleep-related diagnoses, and lifestyle health behaviors. After evaluating for age, body mass index, race, employment status, marital status, level of education, household income, and history or current diagnosis of depression, they found that women with fibromyalgia were more likely to have had reproductive health or sleep-related diagnoses, including premenstrual syndrome, dysmenorrhoea, breast cysts, bladder cystitis, sleep apnea, restless leg syndrome, and abnormal leg movements. They were calculated to use less then half as many calories per week as control women and had more sleep pattern difficulties, lower alcohol use, and more negative changes in sexual function. More specifically, women with fibromyalgia showed significantly decreased sexual arousal and excitement, decreased experience of orgasm, decreased self-pleasuring/ masturbation, increased vaginal tightness during penetration, and increased pain with intercourse. However, sexual desire was not different between patients with fibromyalgia and healthy controls.

Prins et al. [18] examined sexual functioning at the specific phases of the sexual response cycle among women with fibromyalgia. They applied the Questionnaire for screening Sexual Dysfunctions-Short Form (QSD-SF) to 63 premenopausal, heterosexual women with fibromyalgia (age: 21-54 years) who were recruited at meetings of regional patient associations.

The QSD-SF is a multidimensional self-report questionnaire to assess the frequency of and trouble experienced with sexual problems during the past few months. Seventeen scales assess sexual functioning during four phases of the sexual response cycle (desire, excitement, orgasm, and resolution), while six scales assess genital and bodily pain. Frequencies of sexual activities are rated on 7-point (1 = less than once per month, 7 = several times a day) or 5-point Likert-scales (1 = almost never, 5 = always). Five-point Likert scales are also used to assess the experienced trouble (1 = no trouble, 5 = very much trouble) and satisfaction (1 = very dissatisfied, 5 = very satisfied).

They found that women with fibromyalgia reported more problems with typical desire phase sexual activities, while none of the scales of the sexual excitement phase and the sexual orgasm phase showed a difference between patients and the healthy group. At the resolution phase, the women with fibromyalgia reported to be less sexually satisfied than the healthy women. Women with fibromyalgia reported more problems with genital insensitivity, as well as pain in other parts of their body, before, during, or after having sexual contact with their partner, but genital pain did not differ between the groups. Sexual functioning did not differ between patients with or without antidepressants therapy, with the exception of two scales: Mann-Whitney U tests showed that antidepressants went together with excitement and orgasm problems. The group that used anxiolytics reported more sexual dissatisfaction. Regression analysis confirmed that within the group of patients with fibromyalgia, mental distress is associated with sexual dysfunction.

Finally, Orellana et al. [24] studied the prevalence of sexual dysfunction in female patients with fibromyalgia, the impact of fibromyalgia on sexual activity and the factors associated with sexual dysfunction in these patients. They enrolled 31 patients with fibromyalgia, and used as controls 20 aged-matched healthy women and 26 patients with rheumatoid arthritis. It has been shown that patients with rheumatoid arthritis have sexual dysfunction [25].

Sexual function was assessed by the Changes in Sexual Functioning Questionnaire (CSFQ) and a cross-sectional analysis of pain (100-mm VAS scale), anxiety and depression (as determined by the STAI and Beck Depression Inventory scales, respectively) was performed. They found that patients with fibromyalgia and rheumatoid arthritis had a significantly higher rate of sexual dysfunction compared to healthy controls. Sexual dysfunction was more frequent among patients with fibromyalgia (97%) than in patients with rheumatoid arthritis (84%) but without statistical differences. A univariate analysis showed that age (p=0.0002), marital (p=0.036) and work status (p=0.048), pain intensity (p=0.007), level of anxiety (p=0.002), and level of depression (p=0.0005) were significantly associated with sexual dysfunction in fibromyalgia. However, only the intensity of depression was associated with the sexual dysfunction in patients with fibromyalgia in the multivariate analysis (p=0.012).

Additionally, the impact of relationship variables on sexual functioning in women with fibromyalgia has been studied. Kool et al. [26] found that low relationship satisfaction is the strongest and most-frequent predictor of problematic sexual functioning. More fatigue and , more active involvement of the spouse, only after taking account of relationship satisfaction, were associated with reduced sexual functioning and satisfaction. They suggested that for women with fibromyalgia, relationship satisfaction is good for sexual functioning. Although having an involved spouse is good for the relationship, it may be bad for sexual functioning.

IMPACT OF PHYSICAL AND PSYCHOLOGICAL VARIABLES IN SEXUAL FUNCTION IN PATIENTS WITH FIBROMYALGIA: HYPOTHESIS ABOUT THE MECHANISM OF SEXUAL DYSFUNCTION

Sexuality and sexual function are complex aspects of human life, comprising much more than the act of sexual intercourse, involving physical (age, health status, hormonal), psychological (depression, anxiety), and even socio-cultural (religious beliefs) factors [27]. Sexual dysfunction is a multicausal and multidimensional health problem and comprises disease-related factors (biologic and psychosocial components) as well as therapy.

Fibromyalgia is a very common disorder, with a complex physiopathology, possibly including alterations in the neurotransmitters of pain modulation, thalamic perfusion dysfunction, and changes in the hypothalamic–pituitary–adrenal axis [28].

In patients with fibromyalgia, generalized pain, stiffness, fatigue, and poor sleep are the most common and characteristic symptoms. However, patients with fibromyalgia may also report a sensation of swelling in the soft tissues and paresthesias. Depression and mood disorders may also play an important role in the occurrence of fibromyalgia [15,16]. Consequently, fibromyalgia involves multiple, often severe, sensory, somatic, and cognitive manifestations [23].

Several physical and psychological factors have been implicated in the pathogenesis of sexual dysfunction in patients with fibromyalgia. Pain, fatigue and altered autonomic function are among the most important physical factors implicated. Meanwhile, depression (the most important) anxiety, sexual abuse, and low self-esteem are among the psychological factors implicated. However, other factors linked to sexual dysfunction include irritable bladder, vulvodynia, vaginismus, sleep disorders, overall low physical activity, and factors related to the patient's environment (e.g., partner relationship) (Figure 1).

Pain is an antiaphrodisiac [29], and it is difficult to imagine that patients will achieve sexual satisfaction when high levels of pain are experienced. Pain not only limits sexual satisfaction during intercourse but can also negatively influence sexual desire due to the anticipation of pain.

It has been shown that chronic pain can produce sexual dysfunction. However, although chronic widespread pain is the most common characteristic symptom in patients with fibromyalgia, most studies had moderately correlated pain with sexual dysfunction in these patients. In certain patient subgroups, it was found to not be associated with [23], or to play a minor role in, predicting sexual functioning and satisfaction [26]. Tikiz et al. [21] showed that in patients with fibromyalgia, only pain was associated with sexual dysfunction and that the coexistence of major depression had no additional negative effect on sexual function. Orellana et al. [24] showed a level of sexual dysfunction similar to patients with fibromyalgia in patients with RA, even though pain level was significantly higher in the group with fibromyalgia compared with RA patients.

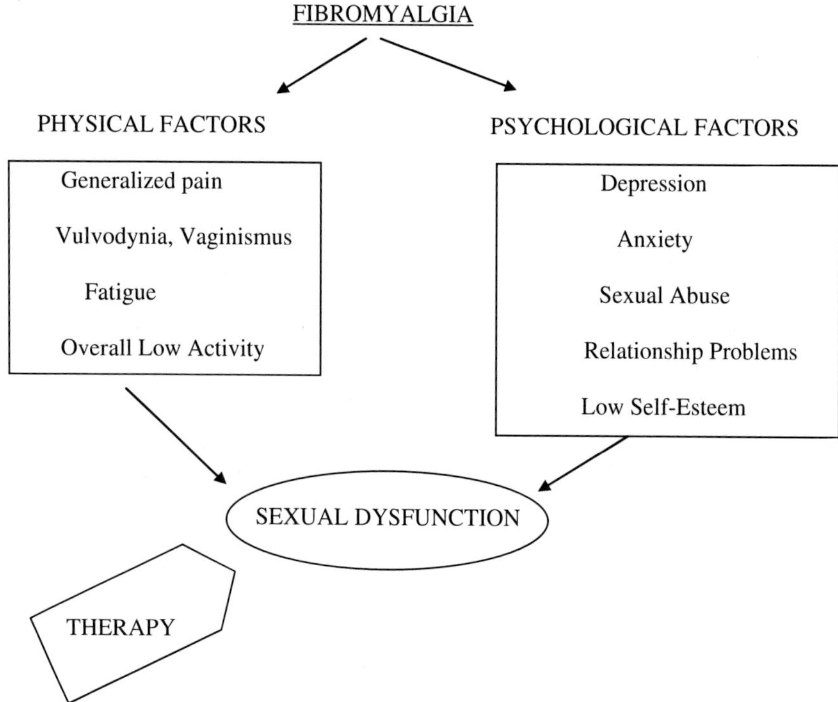

Figure 1. Schematic representation of the factors associated to sexual dysfunction in patients with fibromyalgia.

On the other hand, Prins et al. [18] found a high prevalence of pain in the body before, during and after sex in patients with fibromyalgia but a low prevalence of dyspareunia. They hypothesized that the diffuse, widespread pain of fibromyalgia perhaps does not generalize to pain in the genitals and involves physiological processes other than the local, burning, and sharp pain of dyspareunia. Additionally, there was not an association between pain and psychological aspects of sexuality (excitement and orgasm phases), and surprisingly, more severe pain was even associated with less severe problems in the excitement and orgasm phases. They explained that both pain [30] and the sexual response cycle [31] are under the control of numerous endocrine and central nervous system influences, and neuropeptides that are involved in pain are also involved in sexual behavior.

Also, patients with fibromyalgia have sympathetic hyperactivity with concurrent hyporeactivity, downregulation of β-adrenergic receptors caused by chronic stimulation, and concomitant hypoactivity in the parasympathetic nervous system [32]. Therefore, there could be a relationship between the autonomic nervous system and sexual dysfunctions [33].

Ünlü et al. [34] investigated autonomic dysfunction in patients with fibromyalgia by assessing sympathetic skin response (SSR) from palmar, plantar, and genital regions and evaluated the relation between sexual problems and autonomic dysfunction in these patients. They found that patients with fibromyalgia have a higher prevalence of sexual problems, and the amplitude of SSR recorded from the palmar, plantar, and genital regions was significantly reduced in patients with fibromyalgia compared with age-matched healthy control subjects. However, they did not find any correlation between sexual dysfunction and SSR.

Fatigue is another important symptom in patients with fibromyalgia, but only one study found association between fatigue and sexual dysfunction [26].

Depression, anxiety and other psychiatric and mood disorders are frequently associated with fibromyalgia. Depression is particularly prevalent in patients with fibromyalgia, ranging from 25% to 70% across studies [35]. Depression and anxiety have been cited as possible factors leading to sexual dysfunction in people with chronic pain [36,37]. Also, it has been found that in healthy females, anxiety is associated with reduced frequency of intercourse, whereas depression is an important factor in both loss of libido and loss of sexual satisfaction [38,39].

Aydin et al. [22] found that sexual dysfunction was significantly more frequent in patients with fibromyalgia than in healthy controls, and female sexual function showed a significant negative correlation with depression and anxiety scores. In concordance with that, Orellana et al. [24] showed that only in patients with fibromyalgia was the intensity of depression associated with sexual dysfunction, suggesting that depression plays a major role in this disorder. In contrast, an observational study by Tikiz et al. [21] found that sexual function was significantly decreased in patients with fibromyalgia compared with healthy controls, but no significant difference was found between patients with fibromyalgia only and fibromyalgia plus major depression. They concluded that coexistent major depression had no additional negative effect on sexual function in female patients with fibromyalgia.

Another important issue to be considered is the participation of the antidepressant on sexual dysfunction in patients with fibromyalgia. It has been reported that women receiving selective serotonin reuptake inhibitors often complain of decreased desire, decreased arousal, decreased genital sensation, and difficulty achieving orgasm [40,41]. However, in some studies association between psychiatric medication in patients with fibromyalgia and sexual dysfunction has not been found [24].

Other factors linked to sexual dysfunction include irritable bladder, vulvodynia, vaginismus, sexual abuse, and myofascial tender points [42,43]. Vulvar pain was reported by Gordon et al. [43] in approximately 20.6% of women with fibromyalgia and 16.8% of women with chronic depression in a Web-based study. In concordance with that, Aydin et al. [22] found that complaints of pain during sexual intercourse were more common in patients with fibromyalgia (50%) than in healthy controls (16.7%). Additionally, Shaver et al. [23] found significant association between fibromyalgia and increased pain and vaginal tightness with intercourse. Their hypothesis is that in patients with fibromyalgia the threshold at which sensory input becomes painful is lower than normal, and pain tolerance is low [44], so pain with intercourse is likely.

Some studies have shown that women with chronic pain symptoms more frequently reported a history of sexual abuse or other traumatic events in childhood or adolescence [45,46]. Taylor et al. [47] found sexual abuse in 65% of patients with fibromyalgia; meanwhile Alexander et al. [45] described that 57% of patients with fibromyalgia reported a history of sexual/physical abuse.

The prevalence and type of abuse were not significantly different between groups. Sexually abused subjects with fibromyalgia reported significantly more symptoms than did non-sexually abused women with fibromyalgia, but did not differ in the number of symptoms for which they sought medical treatment [47].

TREATMENT AND RECOMMENDATION

One of the most important issues about the treatment of sexual dysfunction associated with fibromyalgia is the fact that sexual functioning is not routinely addressed by physicians or health professionals, nor is it part of frequently used questionnaires to assess physical function or quality of life. The common problem is communication, so including an open communication inquiry about sexuality into the routine care is the first step to improve the situation. Allowing the patients to present problems and concerns without embarrassment is also important.

After an open communication is achieved, the treatment will depend of the specific patient's symptoms (Table 1). However, there are some general recommendations including discussion of the problems with the partner, principally about the partner's fear in causing pain or distress during sexual intercourse; explores different positions; using analgesic drugs, heat, and muscle relaxants before the sexual activity in order to decrease pain; and exploring alternative methods of sexual expression [48].

In regard to specific treatment, pain and depression are the most important issues. Pain is an antiaphrodisiac [29], and it is difficult to imagine that patients will achieve sexual satisfaction when high levels of pain are experienced. Pain not only limits sexual satisfaction during the intercourse but can also negatively influence sexual desire due to the anticipation of pain. On the other hand, depression is significantly correlated with pain [49], so alleviating pain and controlling depression could break the vicious circle of pain, depression, and sexual dysfunction. For the other specific symptoms, such as dyspareunia due vaginal dryness, the use of vaginal lubricants, estrogen cream and estrogen replacement therapy could be useful (Table 1) [48].

Table 1. Factors Associated With Sexual Dysfunction in Fibromyalgia and Recommendations for Specific Symptoms

Sexual dysfunction	Factors implicated	Recommendations
Sexual disability	Limited mobility	Change position
	Pain, fatigue	Analgesic, heat, and muscle relaxation before activity
Dyspareunia	Vulvodynia, Vaginismus	Vaginal lubrication, estrogen cream.
Diminished desire and	Anxiety, depression	Counseling, antidepresive drugs[a]
Satisfaction	Low self-esteem	

[a] Could decrease libido (Modificated from Tristano 2009, 2011).

REFERENCES

[1] Prady J, Vale A, Hill J. Body image and sexuality. In: Hill J (ed) *Rheumatology nursing: a creative approach*. Churchill Livingstone, Edinburgh, 1998.

[2] Wells D. *Caring for sexuality in health and illness*. Churchill Livingstone, Edinburgh, 2000.

[3] Pitts M. Sexual health. *The psychology of preventative health*. London: Routledge, 1996.

[4] Laumann E, Paik A, and Rosen R. Sexual dysfunction in the United States: prevalence and predictors. *JAMA* 1999;281: 537–544.

[5] Berman JR, and Goldstein I. Female sexual dysfunction. *Urol Clin North Am* 2001;28: 405–416.

[6] Spector IP, and Carey MP. Incidence and prevalence of the sexual dysfunctions: a critical review of the empirical literature.*Arch Sex Behav* 1990;19:389–408.

[7] Sadock VA: Normal human sexuality and sexual and gender identity disorders, in Sadock BJ, and Sadock VA (Eds): *Comprehensive Textbook of Psychiatry*. Philadelphia, Lippincott Williams & Wilkins, 2000, pp 1577–1662.

[8] Basson R, Berman J, Burnett A, Derogatis L, Ferguson D, Fourcroy J, Goldstein I, Graziottin A, Heiman J, Laan E, Leiblum S, Padma-Nathan H, Rosen R, Segraves K, Segraves RT, Shabsigh R, Sipski M, Wagner G, Whipple B. Report of the International Consensus Development Conference on Female Sexual Dysfunction: definitions and classifications. *J Urol* 2000;163:888–893.

[9] Tristano AG. The impact of rheumatic diseases on sexual function. *Rheumatol Int.* 2009 Jun;29(8):853-60.

[10] Ostensen M. New insights into sexual functioning and fertility in rheumatic diseases. *Best Pract Res Clin Rheumatol.* 2004:219-32.

[11] Britto MT, Rosenthal SL, Taylor J, Passo MH. Improving rheumatologists' screening for alcohol use and sexual activity. *Arch Pediatr Adolesc Med* 2000;154(5):478–483

[12] Serrant-Green L. Inequality in provision of sexual health information. *Prof Nurse* 2001;16:1038–42.

[13] Royal College of Nursing. *RCN sexual health strategy. Guidance for nursing staff* (publication code 001 525). London: Royal College of Nursing, 2001.

[14] Wolfe F, Ross K, Anderson J, Russell IJ, Hebert L. The prevalence and characteristics of fibromyalgia in the general population. *Arthritis Rheum.* 1995;38(1):19-28.

[15] Yunus MB, and Inanıcı F: Clinical characteristics and biopathophysiological mechanisms of fibromyalgia syndrome, in Baldry P (Ed): *Myofascial Pain and Fibromyalgia Syndromes: A Clinical Guide to Diagnosis and Management.* Edinburgh, Churchill Livingstone, pp 351–377, 2001.

[16] Yunus MB, and Inanıcı F: Fibromyalgia syndrome: clinical features, diagnosis, and biopathophysiologic mechanisms, in Rachlin ES, and Rachlin I (Eds): *Myofascial Pain and Fibromyalgia:* Trigger Point Management. Philadelphia, Mosby, pp 3–31, 2002.

[17] Ambler N, Williams AC, Hill P, Gunary R, Cratchley G. Sexual difficulties of chronic pain patients. *Clin J Pain.* 2001;17(2):138-45.

[18] Prins MA, Woertman L, Kool MB, Geenen R. Sexual functioning of women with fibromyalgia. *Clin Exp Rheumatol.* 2006;24(5):555-61.

[19] Ryan S, Hill J, Thwaites C, Dawes P. Assessing the effect of fibromyalgia on patients' sexual activity. *Nurs Stand* 2008;23:35– 41.

[20] De Costa ED, Kneubil MC, Leao WC. Assessment of sexual satisfaction in fibromyalgia patients. *Einstein* 2004;2:177– 181.

[21] Tikiz C, Muezzinoglu T, Pirildar T, Taskn EO, Frat A, Tuzun C. Sexual dysfunction in female subjects with fibromyalgia. *J Urol* 2005;174:620– 623.

[22] Aydin G, Basar MM, Keles I, Ergun G, Orkun S, Batislam E. Relationship between sexual dysfunction and psychiatric status in premenopausal women with fibromyalgia. *Urology* 2006;67:156–161.

[23] Shaver JL, Wilbur J, Robinson FP, Wang E, Buntin MS. Women's health issues with fibromyalgia syndrome. *J Womens Health* (Larchmt) 2006;15:1035–1045.

[24] Orellana C, Casado E, Masip M, Galisteo C, Gratacos J, Larrosa M. Sexual dysfunction in fibromyalgia patients. *Clin Exp Rheumatol* 2008;26:663–666

[25] Tristano AG: The Impact of Rheumatic Arthritis on Sexual Function, in Michael H. Madsen (Ed): *Rheumatoid Arthritis: Prevalence, Risk Factors and Health Effects.* NY, NOVA Publishers, pp 137-144, 2011.

[26] Kool MB, Woertman L, Prins MA, Van Middendorp H, Geenen R. Low relationship satisfaction and high partner involvement predict sexual problems of women with fibromyalgia. *J Sex Marital Ther* 2006;32:409–423.

[27]   Kadri N, Mchichi Alami KH, Mechakra Tahiri S. Sexual dysfunction in women: population based epidemiological study. *Arch Womens Ment Health* 2002, 5:59–63.

[28]   Heim C, Ehlert U, Hellhammer DH. The potential role of hypocortisolism in the pathophysiology of stress-related bodily disorders. *Psychoneuroendocrinology* 2000; 25:1–35.

[29]   Ehrlich GE. Social, economic, psychologic, and sexual outcomes in rheumatoid arthritis. *Am J Med* 1983;75:27–34.

[30]   Pillemer SR, Bradley LA, Crofford LJ, Moldofsky H, Chrousos GP. The neuroscience and endocrinology of fibromyalgia. *Arthritis Rheum.* 1997;40(11):1928-39.

[31]   Meston CM, Frohlich PF. The neurobiology of sexual function. *Arch Gen Psychiatry.* 2000;57(11):1012-30.

[32]   Martinez-Lavin M, Hermosillo AG. Autonomic nervous system dysfunction may explain the multisystem features of fibromyalgia. *Semin Arthritis Rheum* 2000, 29:197–199.

[33]   Orellana C, Gratacós J, Galisteo C, Larrosa M. Sexual dysfunction in patients with fibromyalgia.*Curr Rheumatol Rep.* 2009;11(6):437-42.

[34]   Unlü E, Ulaş UH, Gürçay E, Tuncay R, Berber S, Cakçi A, Odabaşi Z. Genital sympathetic skin responses in fi bromyalgia syndrome. *Rheumatol Int* 2006, 26:1025–1030.

[35]   Meyer-Lindenberg A, Gallhofer B. Somatized depression as a subgroup of fi bromyalgia syndrome. *Z Rheumatol* 1998,57:92–93.

[36]   Monga TN, Tan G, Ostermann HJ, Monga U, Grabois M. Sexuality and sexual adjustment of patients with chronic pain. *Disabil Rehabil* 1998;20:317–329.

[37]   Ambler N, Williams AC, Hill P, Gunary R, Cratchley G. Sexual difficulties of chronic pain patients. *Clin J Pain* 2001;17:138–145.

[38]   Channon LD, Ballinger SE. Some aspects of sexuality and vaginal symptoms during menopause and their relation to anxiety and depression. *Br J Med Psychol* 1986;59:173–180

[39]   Frohlich P, Meston C. Sexual functioning and self-reported depressive symptoms among college women. *J Sex Res* 2002;39:321–325.

[40]   Clayton AH. Female sexual dysfunction related to depression and antidepressant medications. *Curr Womens Health Rep* 2002, 2:182–187.

[41]   Montejo AL, Llorca G, Izquierdo JA, Rico-Villademoros F. Incidence of sexual dysfunction associated with antidepressant agents: a prospective multicenter study of 1022 outpatients. Spanish Working

Group for the Study of Psychotropic-Related Sexual Dysfunction. *J Clin Psych* 2001, 62:10–21.

[42] Wallace DJ, Brock J. *Making Sense of Fibromyalgia.* New York: Oxford University Press; 1999.

[43] Gordon AS, Panahian-Jand M, McComb F, Melegari C, Sharp S. Characteristics of women with vulvar pain disorders: responses to a Web-based survey. *J Sex Marital Ther* 2003;29(Suppl 1):45–58.

[44] Bendtsen L, Norregaard J, Jensen R, Olesen J. Evidence of qualitatively altered nociception in patients with fibromyalgia. *Arthritis Rheum* 1997;40:98–102.

[45] Alexander RW, Bradley LA, Alarcon GS, et al.: Sexual and physical abuse in women with fibromyalgia: association with outpatient health care utilization and pain medication usage. *Arthritis Care Res* 1998, 11:102–115.

[46] Castro I, Barrantes F, Tuna M, et al.: Prevalence of abuse in fibromyalgia and other rheumatic disorders at a specialized clinic in rheumatic diseases in Guatemala City. *J Clin Rheumatol* 2005, 11:140–145.

[47] Taylor ML, Trotter DR, Csuka ME: The prevalence of sexual abuse in women with fi bromyalgia. *Arthritis Rheum* 1995, 38:229–234.

[48] Panush RS, Mihailescu GD, Gornisiewicz MT, Sutaria SH, Wallace DJ. Sex and arthritis. *Bull Rheum Dis.* 2000;49(7):1-4.

[49] Abdel-Nasser AM, Abd El-Azim S, Taal E, El-Badawy SA, Rasker JJ, Valkenburg HA. Depression and depressive symptoms in rheumatoid arthritis patients: an analysis of their occurrence and determinants. *Br J Rheumatol* 1998;37:391–397.

In: Fibromyalgia
Editor: Antonio G. Tristano

ISBN: 978-1-62257-678-4
© 2013 Nova Science Publishers, Inc.

Chapter 2

PSYCHIATRIC COMORBIDITY IN PATIENTS WITH FIBROMYALGIA

Andrea Aguglia[1], Virginio Salvi[1], Filippo Bogetto[1], Eugenio Aguglia[2] and Giuseppe Maina[1,]*

[1]Mood and Anxiety Disorders Unit, Department of Neuroscience,
University of Turin, Italy
[2]Department of Biological Chemistry,
Medical Chemistry and Molecular Biology, University of Catania, Italy

ABSTRACT

Fibromyalgia (FM) is a common and polymorphic neurosensory disease, characterized by a condition of chronic and widespread musculoskeletal pain and higher pain perception in specific anatomic sites, called tender points. This illness, of unknown etiology, predominantly affects young or middle-aged women. FM is frequent in the general population and clinical samples: the prevalence has been estimated between 0.5% and 5% in epidemiological studies and up to 15% in clinical samples across different countries. In Italy the reported lifetime prevalence is 2.2%.

Multiple comorbid medical conditions may be associated with fibromyalgia, including tension headache or migraine, irritable bowel syndrome, and non-dermatomal paresthesias. Furthermore, there is

---

[*] Corresponding Author: Prof. Giuseppe Maina. Address: via cherasco 11 - 10121 – Turin. Tel: 0039011/6335425; Fax: 0039011/673473. Email: giuseppemaina@hotmail.com.

mounting data supporting comorbidity of fibromyalgia syndrome with psychiatric symptoms, such as unrefreshing sleep, memory and attention impairment, and syndromes like depression, panic disorder, and post-traumatic stress disorder; these conditions are extremely prevalent, ranging from 20 to 80% in clinical samples of patients with FM. The assessment of psychiatric conditions, in particular depression and anxiety, in patients suffering from FM has important clinical implications with regard to course and severity of illness, quality of life and functional impairment, and treatment response.

In this review we aim at examining the current literature regarding psychiatric comorbidity of FM. We carried out a search on MEDLINE and PUBMED from 1966 to nowadays using the following keywords: fibromyalgia, depression, anxiety, and psychiatric comorbidity. We selected both epidemiological and clinical studies, written in English.

The review will help the audience of clinicians to enhance the understanding of the impact of psychiatric comorbidities on the course and treatment of FM, in order to analyze the combined effect of these two conditions and to optimize patients' long-term outcomes.

INTRODUCTION

Fibromyalgia (FM) is a common and polymorphic neurosensory disease of unknown etiology classified among extra-articular rheumatisms of functional nature. It is characterized by a condition of chronic and widespread musculoskeletal pain and a heightened and painful response to tactile stimuli: as a matter of fact, for diagnosis of FM, the American College of Rheumatology Criteria (ACR) (Wolfe et al., 1990) includes the presence of pain of for at least three months duration in all four body quadrants in combination with excess tenderness to manual palpation in at least eleven or more specific anatomic sites, called "tender points" (18 specific points at 9 bilateral sites) and in the absence of clinically demonstrable peripheral nociceptive causes (Chakrabarty and Zorob, 2007).

In recent years, the evidence that fibromyalgia may be considered a physical illness is increasing. At present, FM appears in the International Statistical Classification of Diseases and Related Health Problems, 10th Revision (ICD-10) (WHO, 1992) under rheumatic diseases, is treated likewise by the International Association for the Study of Pain as a specific physical condition (Merskey, 1994), is accepted by the majority of rheumatologists and family practitioners as a physical diagnosis, and has accumulated impressive positive physical and negative psychological evidence (Merskey et al., 2008).

Other researchers moderately claim that "symptom amplification because of a pathologic misperception of internal stimuli" occurs in FM and encourages patients and physicians to accept that more symptoms of the syndrome are psychological (Wienfiel et al., 2001). These data have been confirmed by other authors such as Shapiro and Netter (Netter et al., 1998; Shapiro et al., 2003).

FM is frequent in population and clinical samples: the prevalence was estimated between 0.5% and 5% in general population studies and up to 15% in clinical samples across different countries (White and Harth, 2001; Neumann and Buskila, 2003). In Italy, the reported lifetime prevalence is 2.2% (Branco et al., 2010). FM is more common in women than in men, affecting the 3.4% of women versus the 0.5% of men (Wolfe et al., 1990). The ratio of women to men affected by FM varies between 9:1 and 20:1 (Schneider, 1995; Burckhardt et al., 1998; Nampiaparampil 2004); therefore, FM predominantly affects women even though it is still not known why there is a massive predilection for the female gender. Patients are usually diagnosed between the ages of 20 and 50 years, and the incidence rises with age so that, by age 80, approximately 8% of adults meet the classification criteria established by the American College of Rheumatology (Wolfe et al., 1997).

Multiple comorbid medical conditions are associated with FM, including tension headache or migraine, irritable bowel syndrome, non-dermatomal paresthesias, colicky abdominal pain, orthostatic hypotension, and dizziness (Solano et al., 2009).

The association between FM and depression appears to be particularly strong (Kassam et al., 2006). Increasing evidence indicates that the relationship between both disorders is bidirectional and that both disorders may be part of an "affective spectrum" of disorders based on the findings of overlapping symptomatology, similar pattern of comorbid disorders, and high rates of depression among relatives of patients with FM (Hudson and Pope, 1996; Haug et al., 2004; Raphaet et al., 2004; Aggarwal et al., 2006; Kanaan et al., 2007; Leiknes et al., 2007; Pae et al., 2008). Depressive symptoms are indeed frequent in patients with FM, with prevalence rates around 40-83% (Kato et al., 2006; Aguglia et al., 2011). Other syndromes like bipolar disorder (BD), generalized anxiety disorder (GAD), panic disorder (PD), and post-traumatic stress disorder (PTSD) are also frequent in patients with FM, ranging from 13 to 80% in clinical samples (Arnold et al., 2008). An Italian study reported that patients with FM showed a higher comorbidity with GAD, PD, and depression than controls: the study showed a high frequency of manic symptoms in the sample of fibromyalgia patients (59%), approximately double that found in the control sample (Carta et al., 2006). Furthermore, there is mounting data supporting comorbidity of fibromyalgia syndrome with psychiatric symptoms, such as unrefreshing sleep, attention and memory impairment.

The assessment of psychiatric conditions, in particular depression and anxiety, in patients suffering from FM has important implications for two reasons: clinical and health care impact. From a clinical point of view, comorbidity between FM and psychiatric disorders affects course and severity of illness, quality of life, functional impairment, and treatment response. For example, the number of reported medical symptoms is positively associated with current and past depressive and anxiety disorders (Walker et al., 1997). On the other hand, high levels of depression and anxiety are associated with more physical symptoms, worse perceived health, interference from pain, and life stress (White et al., 2002). Mood and anxiety disorders are also associated with disability, in terms of a worse quality of life and functioning, in patients with FM (Epstein et al., 1999).

With these premises, the goal of the study is to examine the current literature regarding FM and its psychiatric comorbidities, in order to enhance the understanding of how psychiatric disorders may contribute to abnormal pain sensitivity, worse quality of life and eventually increased health care costs in individuals with FM.

METHODS

In this review we aim at examining the current literature regarding psychiatric comorbidity of FM. A detailed research was performed in PUBMED from 1966 to nowadays using the following keywords: fibromyalgia, depression, anxiety disorder(s), and psychiatric comorbidity. We selected both epidemiological and clinical studies, written in English. Moreover, only papers published in peer-reviewed journals and employing standardized experimental procedures and validated assessment scales have been considered.

THE COMORBIDITY BETWEEN FIBROMYALGIA AND PSYCHIATRIC DISORDERS

A large number of patients with FM have substantial lifetime psychiatric comorbidity. Up to 90% of FM patients, compared with the 17% of the general population, suffer from depression during their lifetime (Wilke et al., 2010) and approximately 18-36% of patients with FM report a current major depressive disorder (MDD) (Marangell et al., 2011). In a prospective study, Forseth and colleagues examined 214 women with self-reported pain in a period between 1990 and 1995. Thirty-nine of these women fulfilled the American College of Rheumatology criteria for FM while the other 175 women that showed a condition of widespread pain were assessed as individuals at risk for developing FM. After five years forty-three (25%) women developed FM. The presence of depression was found to be a strong risk factor for the development of FM (Forseth et al., 1999). Patients with FM display high rates of comorbidity not only with depressive but also with anxiety disorders: their prevalence has been reported in 19-80% and in 12-64% of patients enrolled in clinical studies (Buskila et al., 2007; Fietta et al., 2007; Uguz et al., 2010). The reported high variability could be explained by the different study setting, since most of the studies were carried out in tertiary care settings in which psychiatric disorders can be overrepresented, while other studies were conducted in primary clinical and community settings (Buskila et al., 2007; Fietta et al., 2007). Uguz et al. investigated Axis I and II disorders in a sample of outpatients affected by FM compared with a control group, showing that 48% of patients had an Axis I disorder (Uguz et al., 2010). As already mentioned, the reported rates of comorbidity generally vary greatly: for MDD from 15% to 62% (Thieme et al., 2004; Carta et al., 2006; Kassam et al., 2006; Nordahl et., 2007; Arnold et al., 2008; Ross et al., 2010; Uguz et al., 2010; de Melo Santos et al., 2011; Fiest et al., 2011; Marangell et al., 2011; Schaefer et al., 2011); for BD between 13% and 30% (Carta et al., 2006; Arnold et al., 2008; Wilke et al., 2010); for GAD, social phobia (SP) and PD from 5% and 40%, 8% and 21% and 28%, respectively (Carta et al., 2006; Arnold et al., 2008). Regarding PTSD, in subjects with FM, the expected prevalence is between 8% and 23% (Thieme et al., 2004; Arnold et al., 2008), even though symptoms of PTSD have been reported in 56% of patients with FM (Sherman et al., 2000; Cohen et al., 2002).

Fietta and colleagues postulated three hypotheses to explain the relationship between FM and psychiatric disorders: the first one suggests that psychiatric disorders may be a reaction to the chronic pain and disability of FM patients, but this is inconsistent with the observation that psychiatric disorders may precede the onset of FM and that there is a high rate of them among relatives of FM patients. The second hypothesis assumes that FM is consequent to an underlying psychiatric disorder; however, many patients with FM never develop any psychiatric disorder in their lifetime. The third hypothesis suggests a common biological diathesis between psychiatric disorders and FM, tentatively involving shared alterations in the dopaminergic and serotoninergic transmission (Fietta et al., 2007). In particular, patients with FM have been found to have a higher frequency of the short/short (s/s) genotype of the promoter region of the serotonin transporter compared to healthy controls. The short allele subgroup of patients with FM also showed greater mean levels of depression, anxiety and psychological distress. Finally, the high comorbidity rates between FM and PTSD have been explained by the presence of stressful life events in childhood/adolescence, which are indeed very common in patients with FM (Anderberg et al., 2000). It is possible that the "emotional pain" may be converted into physical pain so that the somatic complaints of FM patients may be in part secondary adaptive mechanisms of avoidance, conditioned by post-traumatic factors. Moreover FM and PTSD could share common pathophysiological factors: some data suggest that relatively low baseline cortisol is associated with the development of PTSD and that in FM there is a hypoactivity of the hypothalamic-pituitary-adrenal (HPA) axis (Buskila et al., 2007).

Concerning Axis II disorders, a recent study conducted by Uguz and coworkers on a sample of 103 patients with FM showed a rate of comorbidity of personality disorders of 31%. The majority of patients were affected by obsessive-compulsive personality disorder (23%), but avoidant and passive-aggressive personality disorders were more frequently identified in the patients' group than in the controls (11% vs. 2%) (Uguz et al., 2010). Another study found that patients with FM had a high prevalence rate of personality disorders, in particular borderline personality disorder (9%) (Thieme et al., 2004). Finally, Rose and colleagues reported that 47% of patients with FM received at least one diagnosis of personality disorder, specifically obsessive-compulsive personality disorder, 30%; borderline personality disorder, 16.7%; and depressive personality disorder, 16.7% (Rose et al., 2009). The data are summarized in table 1.

As previously pointed out, a large range of comorbidities between FM and psychiatric disorders has been reported considering data from different studies; this variability can be due to a variety of different factors including the type of study, the characteristics of the patients' sample and the methods used for diagnostic evaluation. Concerning the type of study, the retrospective investigations can be responsible for errors in reconstructions of patients' history, and this can obviously bias lifetime comorbidity rates. Even the type of control group should be considered: some studies employed healthy controls, while in one the controls for FM patients were patients with rheumatoid arthritis (RA). In fact, it's obvious that anxiety/depressive symptoms/disorders are much more common among non-healthy than among healthy people. The characteristics of the sample can also influence the results, both the age of patients and the numerousness of the sample; indeed the power of statistical analyses can be related to sample size since the results are more reliable as a greater number of subjects are recruited. Even the kind of recruitment should be considered since in most studies patients were recruited from tertiary care settings where they may represent a subset with more severe and treatment-resistant illness, or with a higher frequency of comorbidities than patients managed in primary care clinics. Additionally, it has been suggested that a higher incidence of psychiatric comorbidity characterizes patients with fibromyalgia who actively seek medical care, resulting in ascertainment bias, since people with two disorders seek treatment more often than those with only one disorder (Raphael et al., 2006; Wilke et al., 2010).

Moreover, the presence of a pharmacological therapy and its duration and type play an important role because they can mask symptoms and disturbances. Other factors to consider when interpreting data are cultural differences, the country where the study took place and the socioeconomic class.

THE IMPACT OF PSYCHIATRY COMORBIDITY ON FIBROMYALGIA

The presence of psychiatric comorbidities, particularly mood and anxiety disorders, affects the course and severity of FM. These patients often share a common history that includes circadian disturbances, loss of appetite and libido, and a higher number of reported medical symptoms (MacFarlane et al., 1996).

Some studies conducted in patients with FM have found that the presence of comorbid depression and/or anxiety predicts a worsening of pain perception that causes an increase in reported pain symptoms.

Table 1. Prevalence of Psychiatric Comorbities in Patients with Fibromyalgia in Clinical Sample

Author	N	Psychiatric Disorder	%
Epstein SA et al., 1999	73	Mood Disorder lifetime	69%
		Mood Disorder current	29%
		Anxiety Disorder lifetime	35%
		Anxiety Disorder current	27%
Sherman JJ et al., 2000	93	Post-traumatic Stress Disorder symptoms	56%
Cohen H et al., 2002	77	Post-traumatic Stress Disorder symptoms	57%
Thieme K et al., 2004	115	Axis I disorders	77.3%
		Axis II disorders	8.7%
		Anxiety Disorders	32.2%
		Mood Disorders	34.8%
		Substance-related Disorders	1.8%
		Eating Disorders	1.8%
		Post-traumatic Stress Disorder	7.8%
		Borderline personality disorder	5.3%
		Avoidant personality disorder	1.8%
		Dependent personality disorder	1.8%
Güven AZ et al., 2005	53	Depression	90%
		Mild depression	50%
		Moderate depression	38%
		Severe depression	2%
Carta MG et al., 2006	37	Bipolar Disorder	29.7%
		Major Depressive Disorder	62.2%
		Generalized Anxiety Disorder	40.5%
		Social Phobia	8.1%
		Panic Disorder	27.1%
Kassam A et al., 2006	115160	Major Depression (annual prevalence)	22.2%
Nordahl HS et., 2007	44	Major Depressive Disorder (current)	29.5%
		Major Depressive Disorder (lifetime)	27.3%
Arnold et al., 2008	78	Major Depressive Disorder	62%
		Bipolar I Disorder	1%
		Bipolar II Disorder	12%
		Any Anxiety Disorder	60%
		Panic Disorder	28%
		Post-traumatic Stress Disorder	23%
		Generalized Anxiety Disorder	5%
		Social Phobia	21%
		Obsessive-Compulsive Disorder	6%

Author	N	Psychiatric Disorder	%
Uguz F et al., 2010	103	Major depression	14.6%
		Specific phobia	13.6%
		Avoidant Personality Disorder	10.7%
		Obsessive-compulsive Personality Disorder	23.3%
			10.7%
		Passive-aggressive Personality Disorder	47.6%
		Any Axis I disorder	31.1%
		Any Axis II disorder	
Wilke WS et al., 2010	128	Bipolar Disorder	25.2%
de Melo Santos D et al., 2011	69	Major Depression Episode	40.5%
Fiest KM et al., 2011	15591 (age >50ys)	Major Depression	26.2%
Marangell LB et al., 2011	1411	Major Depressive Disorder	26%
Schaefer C et al., 2011	203	Depressive symptoms	57.6%
		Anxiety	49.8%
		Major Depressive Disorder	23.2%
Koroschetz J et al., 2011	1434	Depressive disorders	92.7%
		Anxiety disorders	17.9%
Ross RL et al., 2011	76	Major Depressive Disorder with atypical features	52.6%
		Major Depressive Disorder with melancholic features	35.6%

Walker and colleagues compared 36 patients with FM to 33 patients with rheumatoid arthritis; the authors found that 90% of the patients with FM had a prior psychiatric diagnosis compared with less than half of the patients with rheumatoid arthritis. Patients with comorbid depression had a higher mean number of medically unexplained physical symptoms across several organ systems (Walker et al., 1997). White et al. compared 74 patients with FM and 48 adults with chronic widespread pain but not FM. Compared to pain controls, patients with FM were more symptomatic on virtually all measures of psychological distress. Furthermore, individuals with FM who scored above cut-off scores for depression and anxiety were associated with more physical symptoms and had poorer functioning compared to subjects without depression and anxiety (White et al., 2002). Aguglia and colleagues conducted a study on 30 patients with FM, finding that the concomitant presence of a depressive syndrome, defined by a Hamilton Rating Depression Scale (HRDS) score $\geq$ 8, increased pain perception as measured by means of the Visual Analogue Scale (VAS) for pain (Aitken, 1969): patients with FM and depression had a significantly higher VAS score of 7.1 versus patients without a depressive syndrome (4.2) (Aguglia et al., 2011). Finally, Jansen and colleagues have studied differences in symptomatology between women on long-term sick-leave with musculoskeletal pain with and without concomitant depression. The authors included 332 female and divided them in four subgroups: low back/joint disorder (n = 150), myalgia (n = 47), FM (n = 87), and depression without somatic pain (n = 52). The authors found that VAS scores were significantly higher in patients with FM and comorbid depression compared with all other groups, with or without concomitant depression. On the contrary, the presence of coexisting depression in patients with myalgia or low back/joint disorder did not influence VAS scores (Jansen et al., 2011).

On the other hand, some studies have investigated the impact of FM on depressive symptoms and sleep function.

Ross and colleagues studied 76 subjects with FM and evaluated the presence of depression. The authors found that 88% of patients had a comorbid major depressive episode: most of them had an episode with atypical features (53%), while the 35% had melancholic features. The duration of FM correlated with the presence of atypical symptoms (Ross et al., 2010). FM also impairs sleep. Affleck and colleagues investigated the temporal sequence of sleep and pain among a sample of patients with FM over a 30-day period, using handheld devices to record sleep quality in the morning and pain throughout the day. Their findings suggest that sleep difficulties the night before predict increased pain during the day after; on the contrary, presence of pain during the day does not predict poorer subsequent sleep (Affleck et al., 1996).

Other authors, employing an actigraph to study increased sleeping during the day, and significantly more sleep interruptions and body movements at night, have been found in patients of FM (Korszun et al., 2002). Vishne and colleagues studied the impact of FM in 84 patients in a major depressive episode and 84 healthy controls. FM was more prevalent among depressed females; 26% versus 2% (p=.002). The presence of FM worsened the quality of sleep, measured by the Sleep History Questionnaire, in women with depression compared with the other groups (Vishne et al., 2008). Finally, other researchers studied 492 subjects with FM who completed a 1-year assessment for pain, depression, and sleep quality (assessed with the Pittsburgh Sleep Quality Index). The authors found that sleep disturbances at baseline predicted greater pain after 1 year. A path analysis also indicated that sleep predicted pain, pain predicted a worse physical functioning, and physical functioning eventually predicted depression after 1 year (Bigatti et al., 2008). Clearly, sleep problems among patients with FM impact symptoms in the long term and deserve more attention, both in research and in clinical practice, because they initiate a cascade of symptoms that may lead to depression.

The comorbidity between FM and psychiatric disorders also increases health care costs. A study conducted in the United States using administrative health care and disability claims data compared the economic burden associated with co-morbid depression and FM. The authors demonstrated that both direct costs (due to medical services) and indirect costs (primarily due to absenteeism) were higher in patients with FM and comorbid depression than patients with any single condition. In particular, patients with FM plus depression cost $11,899 per working year, versus $8,073 and $5,163 for employees with depression and FM alone, respectively (Robinson et al., 2004).

SUICIDE AND MORTALITY

The cardinal symptom of FM syndrome is chronic and widespread pain, worsening overall functioning and quality of life. Furthermore, depressive disorder and symptoms are frequently associated with FM. Therefore, it is not surprising that FM is associated with increased risk of suicide than the general population. The assessment of suicide prevalence and predictors in these patients is of outstanding clinical relevance.

Tang and Crane carried out a systematic review to identify, among patients with FM and chronic pain, potential risk factors for suicide. Twelve relevant articles examining suicide, suicide attempts, and suicidal ideation were included in the review. The lifetime prevalence of suicide attempts was between 5% and 14% in individuals with FM and chronic pain, with the prevalence of suicidal ideation being approximately 20%. Eight risk factors for suicidality in chronic pain were identified: comorbid depression, family history of suicide, previous suicide attempt, female sex, and pain-related factors such as type, intensity and duration of pain, and pain-associated insomnia (Tang and Crane, 2006).

More recently, Ratcliffe and colleagues conducted an epidemiologic prospective study on the Canadian population (N=36,984), studying the correlation between chronic pain conditions (FM, back problems, migraine, and arthritis) and suicidal ideation and attempts. The prevalence of migraine, arthritis, back problems, and FM were 10.7%, 17.5%, 20.9%, and 1.5%, respectively. The authors found a positive association between 1 or more chronic pain conditions and suicide ideation (OR=1.46) and attempts (OR=1.94). Patients with FM had an increased risk for suicide attempts; however, after adjusting for the presence of comorbid mood, anxiety or substance use disorders, the association was no more statistically significant: the association between FM and suicide was then due to the comorbid mental disorders (Ratcliffe et al., 2008).

In a recent study, Dreyer and coworkers analyzed the causes of mortality in a large cohort of 1,353 Danish patients with FM, most of which were women. A significantly increased risk of death from suicide was observed in all female patients, with a 10-fold risk of death for suicide in women with FM versus the general population. The excess mortality from suicide in patients with confirmed FM remained the same over time: at the time of diagnosis, the mortality ratio was 6.6, and after 5 years it was 8.2. In contrast with the other studies, none of the patients with FM who committed suicide had a history of depression or other psychiatric disorder at the time of diagnosis. The authors concluded that the increased risk for suicide might be carried by pain itself, fatigue, together with physiological abnormalities, such as increased sympathetic activity or increases in interleukin-10 concentration (Dreyer et al., 2010).

Finally, Calandre and colleagues have conducted a concise survey in 795 Spanish patients, of which only 180 returned the questionnaire. The survey was performed to evaluate the prevalence of previous suicide attempts (as measured through the Plutchik suicide risk scale) in patients with FM and its potential relationship with socio-demographic and clinical characteristics of the disease. Comorbidity was frequent: patients had a mean of 1.19 for mental disorder, particularly depression and anxiety. Thirty (16.7%) patients, all of them women, reported previous suicide attempts. A strong positive correlation was found between the severity of FM and suicide risk: patients with a lifetime suicide attempt had higher scores at the Revised Fibromyalgia Impact Questionnaire (FIQR) versus those without a suicide attempt (76.3 vs 64.3). Again, the association between FM symptoms and suicide risk was driven by the presence of psychiatric symptoms such as depression, anxiety, and poor sleep quality, while pain scores alone were not significantly different among suicide attempters and non-attempters, again confirming the key role of depression and anxiety in increasing the risk of suicide in FM patients (Calandre et al., 2011).

In conclusion, patients with FM are at increased risk of suicide attempts. The heightened risk seems strongly related to the presence of psychiatric comorbidity, in particular depression and anxiety disorders.

QUALITY OF LIFE

Quality of life is somewhat difficult to define, depending on the scale of assessment chosen by the clinician, but also on the emotional and personal resources of each one. More specifically, Health Related Quality of Life (HRQoL), or perceived health, includes those aspects of life that are directly related to physical and mental functioning and with the state of well-being (Guyatt et al., 1993).

The FM is a chronic painful process, which may cause significant limitations in daily life activities. In addition, recently, researchers have showed an increased interest in the evaluation of quality of life in patients with a diagnosis of FM; indeed, there are some evidences that HRQoL is often affected in these patients. FM is often associated with mental illness, as shown before: the presence of psychiatric conditions during clinical presentation negatively influences the quality of life of patients with FM (Gonzales et al., 2010).

Several studies found that quality of life is worsened in FM patients (Neumann et al., 2000; Martinez et al., 2001; Pagano et al., 2004; Birtane et al., 2007; Hoffman and Dukes, 2008; Tander et al., 2008; Arnold et al., 2009; Gormsen et al., 2010). Furthermore, some studies have reported that this effect might not only be mediated by chronic pain, but also by the presence of depressive symptoms (Tander et al., 2008; Gormsen et al., 2010; Aguglia et al., 2011; Campos and Rodriguez Vasquez, 2011; Jansen et al., 2011; Schaefer et al., 2011). In the first study, the authors compared quality of life scores in 30 patients with FM, 30 with RA, and 30 controls. All domains of quality of life were worse in FM patients than controls, and even worse than RA in the domains of physical role, social functioning, and bodily pain; depressive symptoms strongly correlated with the worse quality of life in FM patients (Tander et al., 2008). In a similar study, Gormsen and colleagues compared 28 patients with FM, 30 with neuropathic pain, and 26 controls. Both FM patients and patients with neuropathic pain had similar pain intensities; however, FM patients displayed a worse role function, general health, vitality, social function, and mental health, which was related to the presence of significant depressive symptoms (Gormsen et al., 2010). Our study, conducted on 30

Italian patients with FM, showed that patients with FM and comorbid depressive symptoms displayed a worse quality of life compared to patients suffering from FM alone (Aguglia et al., 2011). In another study, conducted on 76 adult Portuguese women with FM, female patients with FM experienced the maximum influence of their disease on physical dimensions, particularly physical functioning, physical role, general health, and bodily pain, which is consistent with data reported in the literature. Furthermore, anxiety was a significant predictor of a lower score in mental and general health measured by the SF-36, while depression was related with lower scores on vitality and mental health (Campos and Rodriguez Vasquez, 2011). These data have been confirmed by the abovementioned study by Jansen and colleagues, in which HRQoL was evaluated in patients suffering from low back joint disorders (n=150), myalgia (n=43) and FM (n=87), with or without depression. FM and comorbid depression was associated with a lower quality of life in dimensions such as vitality, social functioning, emotional role, and mental health. Furthermore, patients with FM and depression had more difficulties with household tasks such as "peeling potatoes," "washing up by hand," "hanging washing up to dry," and "vacuuming." Patients with FM and depression also had increased difficulties with self-care, particularly with items such as "washing hair" and "brushing hair" (Jansen et al., 2011). A last study divided patients with FM into three groups according to severity of illness (mild, moderate, severe). Severe FM was correlated with depressive and anxiety symptoms (Schaefer et al., 2011). All these studies indicate that coexisting depression decreases HRQoL in several dimensions, particularly regarding mental health.

In conclusion, since depressive symptoms are associated with increased pain perception and worsened quality of life, they must be screened and properly treated in order to improve the pain symptomatology, as well as the quality of life of these patients.

TREATMENT

FM syndrome is the most frequent cause of generalized pain; it is very difficult to treat and it needs a multidisciplinary approach. The therapeutic strategies include antidepressants to treat both pain symptoms and comorbid anxious and depressive symptoms, and use, as needed, of analgesic and anti-inflammatory drugs to decrease pain. Other non-pharmacologic strategies include aerobic exercise, relaxation techniques and psychotherapy, such as

(65% vs. 45%), although the difference did not reach statistical significance. However, the reduction of FIQR scores was significantly greater in depressed (21.1) than in non-depressed patients (41.4). The authors concluded that antidepressant treatment in fibromyalgia was effective in patients with and without major depression, but the functional response was greater in depressed patients (Diaz-Marsa et al., 2011).

Finally, Pae and colleagues, analyzing the possible role of a history of depressive and/or anxiety disorders as a negative predictor of treatment response in patients with FM, found that subjects with or without history of depression and/or anxiety were equally likely to respond to paroxetine CR (response rates: 45.5% vs 37.7% respectively) (Pae et al., 2009).

Some other researchers conducted small studies to assess the efficacy of non-antidepressive treatments in patients with FM with or without comorbid depression. The authors observed that, when treating FM with treatments such as bio-feedback, aerobic exercise, and applied relaxation, the presence of depressive symptoms correlated with non-response to treatment (Ferraccioli et al., 1987; Finset et al., 2004).

Taken all together, these studies strongly suggest the need to treat patients with FM and comorbid psychiatric disorders with treatments effective on both conditions, probably due to the detrimental and independent effect of depression on pain perception.

CONCLUSION

From a critical literature review, it is known that there is a strict association between FM and psychiatric conditions, in particular with depressive and/or anxiety disorders; these patients are also at risk for suicidal behavior. Moreover, as it has been described in the literature, psychiatric comorbidities have a negative impact on the severity and course of pain symptoms of FM, further leading to a poorer quality of life.

Presently, the Outcome Measures in Rheumatology Clinical Trials (OMERACT) workgroup on FM has identified several clinical domains that should be considered when designing clinical trials assessing FM treatments; the identified domains included symptoms not strictly related to FM but commonly prevalent in these patients, such as depression, anxiety, and sleep problems (Mease et al., 2005; Perrot et al., 2010).

In conclusion, the assessment of depression, anxiety, and sleep should be included in the routine diagnostics of FM as well as the presence of widespread pain and the number of tender points. Treatment should focus both on FM and on the symptoms related to comorbid psychiatric disorders.

REFERENCES

Affleck G, Urrows S, Tennen H, Higgins P, Abeles M. Sequential daily relations of sleep, pain intensity, and attention to pain among women with fibromyalgia. *Pain* 1996; 68(2-3): 363-368.

Aggarwal VR, McBeth J, Zakrzewska JM, Lunt M, Macfarlane GJ. The epidemiology of chronic syndromes that are frequently unexplained: do they have common associated factors? *Int J Epidemiol* 2006; 35: 468-476.

Aguglia A, Salvi V, Maina G, Rossetto I, Aguglia E. Fibromyalgia and depressive symptoms: comorbidity and clinical correlates. *J Affect Disorder* 2011; 128: 262-266.

Aitken RCB. Measurement of feelings using visual analogue scales. *Proc Royal Soc Med* 1969; 62: 989.

American Psychiatric Association. Diagnostic and statistical manual for mental disorders. 4th ed. Text Revision. Washington, DC: American Psychiatric Association, 2000.

Amital D, Fostick L, Polliack ML, Segev S, Zohar J, Rubinow A, et al. Posttraumatic stress disorder, tenderness, and fibromyalgia syndrome: are they different entities? *J Psychosom Res* 2006; 61(5): 663-669.

Anderberg UM, Marteins Dottir I, Theorell T, Von Knorring L. The impact of life events in female patients with fibromyalgia and in female healthy controls. *Eur Psychiatry* 2000; 15: 295-301.

Arnold LM, Hess EV, Hudson JI, Welge JA, Berno SE, Keck PE Jr. A randomized, placebo-controlled, double-blind, flexibledose study of fluoxetine in the treatment of women with fibromyalgia. *Am J Med* 2002; 112: 191-197.

Arnold LM, Lu Y, Crofford LJ, Wohlreich M, Detke MJ, Iyengar S, et al. A double-blind, multicenter trial comparing duloxetine with placebo in the treatment of fibromyalgia patients with or without major depressive disorder. *Arthritis Rheum* 2004; 50(9): 2974-2984.

Arnold LM, Rosen A, Pritchett YL, D'Souza DN, Goldstein DJ, Iyengar S, et al. A randomized, double-blind, placebo-controlled trial of duloxetine in the treatment of women with fibromyalgia with or without major depressive disorder. *Pain* 2005; 119: 5-15.

Arnold LM. Management of fibromyalgia and comorbid psychiatric disorders. *J Clin Psychiatry* 2008; 69: 14-19.

Arnold LM, Hudson JI, Wang F, Wohlreich MM, Prakash A, Kajdasz DK, et al. Comparisons of the efficacy and safety of duloxetine for the treatment of fibromyalgia in patients with versus without major depressive disorder. *Clin J Pain* 2009; 25: 461-468.

Arnold LM, Leon T, Whalen E, Barrett J. Relationships among pain and depressive and anxiety symptoms in clinical trials of pregabalin in fibromyalgia. *Psychosomatics* 2010; 51: 489-497.

Bigatti SM, Hernandez AM, Cronan TA, Rand KL. Sleep disturbances in fibromyalgia syndrome: relationship to pain and depression. *Arthritis Rheum* 2008; 59(7): 961-967.

Birtane M, Uzunca K, Tastekin N, Tuna H. The evaluation of quality of life in fibromyalgia syndrome: a comparison with rheumatoid arthritis by using SF-36 health survey. *Clin Rheumatol* 2007; 26: 679-684.

Branco JC, Bannwarth B, Failde I, Abello Carbonell J, Blotman F, Spaeth M, et al. Prevalence of Fibromyalgia: A Survey in Five European Countries. *Semin Arthritis Rheum* 2010; 39(6): 448-453.

Burckhardt CS, Jones KD, Clark SR. Soft tissue problems associated with rheumatic disease. *Lippincotts Prim Care Pract* 1998; 2: 20-29.

Burckhardt CS, Goldenberg D, Crofford L, Gerwin R, Gowans S, Kackson, et al. Guideline for the management of fibromyalgia syndrome. Pain in adults and children. APS Clinical Practice Guideline Series No. 4. Glenview, IL: American Pain Society; 2005.

Buskila D, Cohen H. Comorbidity of fibromyalgia and psychiatric disorders. *Curr Pain Head Rep* 2007; 11: 333-338.

Calandre EP, Vilchez JS, Molina-Barea R, Tovar MI, Garcia-Leiva JM, Hidalgo J, et al. Suicide attempts and risk *Rheumatology (Oxford)* 2011; 50(10): 1889-1893.

Campos RP, Rodriguez Vázquez MI. Health-related quality of life in women with fibromyalgia: clinical and psychological factors associated. *Clin Rheumatol* 2011 (Epub ahead of print).

Carta MG, Cardia C, Mannu F, Intilla G, Hardoy MC, Anedda C, et al. The high frequency of manic symptoms in fibromyalgia does influence the choice of treatment? *Clin Pract Epidemol Ment Health* 2006; 2: 36-41.

Carville SF, Arendt-Nielsen S, Bliddal H, Blotman F, Branco JC, Buskila D, et al. EULAR evidence-based recommendations for the management of fibromyalgia syndrome. *Ann Rheum Dis* 2008; 67: 536-541.

Chakrabarty S, Zoorob R. Fibromyalgia. *Am Fam Physician* 2007; 76(2): 247-254.

Chappell AS, Bradley LA, Wiltse C, Detke MJ, D'Souza DN, Spaeth M. A six-month double-blind, placebo-controlled, randomized clinical trial of duloxetine for the treatment of fibromyalgia. *Int J Gen Med* 2008; 1: 91-102.

Cohen H, Neumann L, Haiman Y, Matar MA, Press J, Buskila D. Prevalence of post-traumatic stress disorder in fibromyalgia patients: overlapping syndromes or post-traumatic fibromyalgia syndrome? *Semin Arthritis Rheum* 2002; 32(1): 38-50.

de Melo Santos D, Lage LV, Kehl Jabur E, Kaziyama HHS, Iosifescu DV, Souza de Lucia MC, et al. The association of major depressive episode and personality traits in patients with fibromyalgia. *Clinics* 2011; 66(6): 973-978.

Díaz-Marsá M, Palomares N, Morón MD, Tajima K, Fuentes ME, López-Ibor JJ, et al. Psychological factors affecting response to antidepressant drugs in fibromyalgia. *Psychosomatics* 2011; 52(3): 237-244.

Dreyer L, Kendall S, Danneskiold-Samsøe B, Bartels EM, Bliddal H. Mortality in a cohort of danish patients with fibromyalgia increased frequency of suicide. *Arthritis Rheum* 2010; 62: 3101-3108.

Epstein SA, Kay G, Clauw D, Heaton R, Klein D, Krupp L, et al. Psychiatric disorders in patients with fibromyalgia. A multicenter investigation. *Psychosomatics* 1999; 40: 57-63.

Ferraccioli G, Ghirelli L, Scita F, Nolli M, Mozzani M, Fontana S, et al. EMG-biofeedback training in fibromyalgia syndrome. *J Rheumatol* 1987; 14(4): 820-825.

Fiest KM, Currie SR, Williams JVA, Wang J. Chronic conditions and major depression in community-dwelling older adults. *J Affect Disord* 2011; 131: 172-178.

Fietta P, Fietta P, Manganelli P. Fibromyalgia and psychiatric disorders. *Acta Biomed* 2007; 78: 88-95.

Finset A, Hørven Wigers S, Götestam KG. Depressed mood impedes pain treatment response in patients with fibromyalgia. *J Rheumatol* 2004; 31: 976-980.

Forseth KO, Førre O, Gran JT. A 5.5 year prospective study of self-reported musculoskeletal *Clin Rheumatol* 1999; 18(2): 114-121.

Fraguas R Jr, Henriques SG Jr, De Lucia MS, Iosifescu DV, Schwartz FH, Menezes PR, et al. The detection of depression in medical setting: a study with PRIME-MD. *J Affect Disord* 2006; 91: 11-17.

Gendreau RM, Thorn MD, Gendreau JF, Kranzler JD, Ribeiro S, Gracely RH, et al. Efficacy of milnacipran in patients with fibromyalgia. *J Rheumatol* 2005; 32: 1975-1985.

Gormsen L, Rosenberg R, Bach FW, Jensen TS. Depression, anxiety *Eur J Pain* 2010; 14(2): 127.

González E, Elorza J, Failde I. Fibromyalgia and psychiatric comorbidity: their effect on the quality of life patients. *Actas Esp Psiquiatr* 2010; 38(5): 295-300.

Gur A, Karakoc M, Nas K, Cevik R, Sarac J, Ataoglu S. Effects of low power laser and low dose amitriptyline therapy on clinical symptoms and quality of life in fibromyalgia: a singleblind, placebo-controlled trial. *Rheumatol Int* 2002; 22: 188-193.

Guyatt GH, Feeny DH, Patrick DL. Measuring health-related quality of life. *Ann Intern Med* 1993; 118: 622-629.

Hannonen P, Malminiemi K, Yli-Kerttula U, Isomeri R, Roponen P. A randomized, double-blind, placebo-controlled study of moclobemide and amitriptyline in the treatment of fibromyalgia in females without psychiatric disorder. *Br J Rheumatol* 1998; 37: 1279-1286.

Haug TT, Mykletun A, Dahl AA. The association between anxiety, depression, and somatic symptoms in a large population: the HUNT-II study. *Psychosom Med* 2004; 66: 845-851.

Häuser W, Thieme K, Turk DC. Guidelines on the management of fibromyalgia syndrome: a systematic review. *Eur J Pain* 2010; 14: 5-10.

Hoffman DL, Dukes EM. The health status burden of people with fibromyalgia: a review of studies that assessed health status with the SF-36 or the SF-12. *Int J Clin Pract* 2008; 62(1): 115-126.

Hudson JI, Pope HG, Jr. The relationship between fibromyalgia and major depressive disorder. *Rheum Dis Clin North Am* 1996; 22: 285-303.

Jansen GB, Linder J, Ekholm KS, Ekholm J. Differences in symptoms, functioning, and quality of life between women on long-term sick-leave with musculoskeletal pain with and without concomitant depression. *J Multidiscip Healthc* 2011; 4: 281-292.

Kanaan RA, Lepine JP, Wessely SC. The association or otherwise of the functional somatic syndromes. *Psychosom Med* 2007; 69: 855-859.

Kassam A, Patten SB. Major depression, fibromyalgia and labour force participation: a population-based cross-sectional study. *BMC Musculoskelet Disord* 2006; 7: 4.

Kato K, Sullivan PF, Evengard B, Pedersen NL. Importance of genetic influences on chronic widespread pain. *Arthritis Rheum* 2006; 54: 1682-1686.

Korszun A, Young EA, Engleberg NC, Brucksch CB, Greden JF, Crofford LA. Use of actigraphy for monitoring sleep and activity level *J Psychosom Res* 2002; 52(6): 439-443.

Leiknes KA, Finset A, Moum T, Sandanger I. Current somatoform disorders in Norway: prevalence, risk factors and comorbidity with anxiety, depression and musculoskeletal disorders. *Soc Psychiatry Psychiatr Epidemiol* 2007; 42: 698-710.

MacFarlane GJ, Thomas E, Papageorgiou AC, Schollum J, Croft PR, Silman AJ. The natural history *J Rheumatol* 1996; 23(9): 1617-1620.

Marangell LB, Clauw DJ, Choy E, Wang F, Shoemaker S, Bradley L, et al. Comparative pain and mood effects in patients with comorbid fibromyalgia and major depressive disorder: Secondary analyses of four pooled randomized controlled trials of duloxetine. *Pain* 2011; 152: 31-37.

Martinez JE, Barauna Filho IS, Kubokawa K, Pedreira IS, Machado LA, Cevasco G. Evaluation *Disabil Rehabil* 2001; 23(2): 64-68.

Mease PJ, Clauw DJ, Arnold LM, Goldenberg DL, Witter J, Williams DA, et al. Fibromyalgia syndrome *J Rheumatol* 2005; 32(11): 2270-2277.

Merskey H, Bogduk N. Classification of chronic pain: descriptions of chronic pain syndromes and definitions of pain terms. 2nd ed. Seattle, Wash: IASP Press; 1994.

Merskey H. Social Influences on the concept of fibromyalgia. *CNS Spectr* 2008; 13 (Suppl 5): 18-21.

Nampiaparampil DE, Shmerling RH. A review of fibromyalgia. *Am J Manag Care* 2004; 10: 794-800.

Netter P, Hennig J. The fibromyalgia syndrome as a manifestation of neuroticism? *Z Rheumatol* 1998; 57: 105-108.

Neumann L, Berzak A, Buskila D. Measuring health *Semin Arthritis Rheum* 2000; 29(6): 400-408.

Neumann L, Buskila D. Epidemiology of fibromyalgia. *Curr Pain Headache Rep* 2003; 7: 362-368.

Nordahl HM, Stiles T. Personality styles in patients with fibromyalgia, major depression and healthy controls. *Ann Gen Psychiatry* 2007; 6: 9.

Norregaard J, Volkmann H, Danneskiold-Samsoe B. A randomized controlled trial of citalopram in the treatment of fibromyalgia. *Pain* 1995; 61: 445-449.

O'Malley PG, Balden E, Tomkins G, Santoro J, Kroenke K, Jackson JL. Treatment of fibromyalgia with antidepressants: a meta-analysis. *J Gen Intern Med* 2000; 15: 659-666.

Ozerbil O, Okudan N, Gokbel H, Levendoglu F. Comparison of the effects of two antidepressants on exercise performance fibromyalgia syndrome and antidepressant treatment 1297 of the female patients with fibromyalgia. *Clin Rheumatol* 2006; 25: 495-497.

Pae CU, Luyten P, Marks DM, Han C, Park SH, Patkar AA, et al. The relationship between fibromyalgia *Curr Med Res Opin* 2008; 24(8): 2359-2371.

Pae CU, Masand PS, Marks DM, Krulewicz S, Peindl K, Mannelli P, et al. History of depressive and/or anxiety disorders as a predictor of treatment response: a post hoc analysis of a 12-week, randomized, double-blind, placebo-controlled trial of paroxetine controlled release in patients with fibromyalgia. *Progr Neuro-Psychopharmacol Biol Psychiatry* 2009; 33: 996-1002.

Pagano T, Matsutani LA, Ferreira EA, Marques AP, Pereira CA. Assessment of anxiety and quality of life in fibromyalgia patients. *Sao Paulo Med J* 2004; 122(6): 252-258.

Patkar AA, Masand PS, Krulewicz S, Mannelli P, Peindl K, Beebe KL, et al. A randomized, controlled, trial of controlled release paroxetine in fibromyalgia. *Am J Med* 2007; 120(5): 448-454.

Perrot S, Winkelmann A, Dukes E, Xu X, Schaefer C, Ryan K, et al. Characteristics of patients with fibromyalgia in France and Germany. *Int J Clin Pract* 2010; 64(8): 1100-1108.

Raphael KG, Janal MN, Nayak S, Schwartz JE, Gallagher RM. Familial aggregation of depression in fibromyalgia: a community-based test of alternate hypotheses. *Pain* 2004; 110: 449-460.

Raphael KG, Malvin N, Janal MN, Nayak S, Joseph E, Schwartz JE, et al. Psychiatric comorbidities in a community sample of women with fibromyalgia. *Pain* 2006; 124: 117-125.

Ratcliffe GE, Enns MW, MD, Belik SL, Sareen J. Chronic pain conditions and suicidal ideation and suicide attempts: an epidemiologic perspective. *Clin J Pain* 2008; 24: 204-210.

Robinson RL, Birnbaum HG, Morley MA, Sisitsky T, Greenberg PE, Wolfe F. Depression and fibromyalgia: treatment and cost when diagnosed separately or concurrently. *J Rheumatol* 2004; 31: 1621-1629.

Rose S, Cottencin O, Chouraki V, Wattier JM, Houvenagel E, Vallet B, et al. Study on personality and psychiatric disorder in fibromyalgia. *Presse Med* 2009; 38(5): 695-700.

Ross RL, Jones KD, Ward RL, Wood LJ, Bennett RM. Atypical depression is more common than melancholic in fibromyalgia: an observational cohort study. *BMC Musculoskeletal Disord* 2010; 11: 120.

Russell J, Mease PJ, Smith TR, Kajdasz DK, Wohlreich MM, Detke MJ, et al. Efficacy and safety of duloxetine for treatment of fibromyalgia in patients with or without major depressive disorder: Results from a 6-month, randomized, double-blind, placebo-controlled, fixed-dose trial. *Pain* 2008; 136: 432-444.

Schaefer C, Chandran A, Hufstader M, Baik R, McNett M, Goldenberg D, et al. The comparative burden of mild, moderate and severe Fibromyalgia: results from a cross-sectional survey in the United States. *Health Qual Life Outcomes* 2011, 9: 71.

Schneider MJ. Tender points/fibromyalgia vs. trigger points/myofascial pain syndrome: a need for clarity in terminology and differential diagnosis. *J Manipulative Physiol Ther* 1995; 18: 398-406.

Shapiro B. Building bridges between body and mind: the analysis of an adolescent with paralyzing chronic pain. *Int J Psychoanal* 2003; 84: 547-561.

Sherman JJ, Turk DC, Okifuji A. Prevalence and impact of posttraumatic stress disorder-like symptoms on patients with fibromyalgia syndrome. *Clin J Pain* 2000; 16(2): 127-134.

Solano C, Martinez A, Becerril L, Vargas A, Figueroa J, Navarro C, et al. Autonomic dysfunction in fibromyalgia *J Clin Rheumatol* 2009; 15(4): 172-176.

Tander B, Cengiz K, Alayli G, Ilhanli I, Canbaz S, Canturk F. A comparative evaluation of health *Rheumatol Int* 2008; 28(9): 859-865.

Tang NK, Crane C. Suicidality in chronic pain *Psychol Med* 2006; 36(5): 575-586.

Thieme K, Turk DC, Flor H. Comorbid depression and anxiety in fibromyalgia syndrome: relationship to somatic and psychosocial variables. *Psychosom Med* 2004; 66: 837-844.

Uceyler N, Hauser W, Sommer C. A systematic review on the effectiveness of treatment with antidepressants in fibromyalgia syndrome. *Arthritis Rheum* 2008; 59(9): 1279-1298.

Uguz F, Çiçek E, Salli A, Karahan AY, Albayrak I, Kaya N, Uğurlu H. Axis I and Axis II psychiatric disorders in patients with fibromyalgia. *Gen Hosp Psychiatry* 2010; 32: 105-107.

Vishne T, Fostick L, Silberman A, Kupchick M, Rubinow A, Amital H, et al. Fibromyalgia among major depression disorder females compared to males. *Rheumatol Int* 2008; 28: 831-836.

Vitton O, Gendreau M, Gendreau J, Kranzler J, Rao SG. A double-blind placebo-controlled trial of milnacipran in the treatment of fibromyalgia. *Hum Psychopharmacol* 2004; 19: 27-35.

Walker EA, Keegan D, Gardner G, Sullivan M, Katon WJ, Bernstein D. Psychosocial factors in fibromyalgia compared with rheumatoid arthritis: I. Psychiatric diagnoses and functional disability. *Psychosom Med* 1997; 59: 565-571.

Wang F, Ruberg SJ, Gaynor PJ, Heinloth AN, Arnold LM. Early improvement in pain *J Pain* 2011; 12(10): 1088-1094.

White KP, Harth M. Classification, epidemiology *Curr Pain Headache Rep* 2001; 5(4): 320-329.

White KP, Nielson WR, Harth M, Ostbye T, Speechley M. Chronic widespread musculoskeletal pain with or without fibromyalgia: psychological distress in a representative community adult sample. *J Rheumatol* 2002; 29: 588-594.

Wilke WS, Gota CE, Muzina DJ. Fibromyalgia and bipolar disorder: a potential problem? *Bipolar Disord* 2010; 12: 514-520.

Winfield JB. Does pain in fibromyalgia reflect somatization? *Arthritis Rheum* 2001; 44(4): 751-753.

Wolfe F, Anderson J, Harkness D, et al. A prospective, longitudinal, multicenter study of service utilization and costs in fibromyalgia. J Am Coll Rheumatol 1997; 40: 1560-1570.

Wolfe F, Smythe HA, Yunus MB, Bennett RM, Bombardier C, Goldenberg DL, et al. The American College of Rheumatology 1990 criteria for the classification of fibromyalgia. Report of the Multicenter Criteria Committee. *Arthritis Rheum* 1990; 33: 160-172.

World Health Organization. The ICD-10 classification of mental and behavioural disorders. Geneva: World Health Organization, 1992.

In: Fibromyalgia
Editor: Antonio G. Tristano

ISBN: 978-1-62257-678-4
© 2013 Nova Science Publishers, Inc.

Chapter 3

EFFECTS OF FIBROMYALGIA IN DENTAL HEALTH

Jordi Ferré-Corominas
University of Barcelona, Oral Medicine Department,
Faculty of Dentistry, Barcelona, Spain

INTRODUCTION

Fibromyalgia is a rheumatic syndrome characterized by chronic musculoskeletal pain, muscle stiffness, sleeping disorders and fatigue. Diagnosis is based on a history of widespread pain and fatigue, which the patient must feel in at least 11 of 18 trigger points for at least three months.

Because of its signs and symptoms, it may be related to other rheumatic conditions like lupus erythematosus, chronic fatigue syndrome, lack of vitamin D or Sjögren Syndrome. Differential diagnosis is very important because prognosis and treatment are different for every patient. Each of these conditions have different signs and symptoms in the oral cavity.

Between 2 and 4% of the population could be diagnosed as having fibromyalgia because their symptoms fit the criteria of the American College of Rheumatology (ACR). It is most common in females between 45 and 60.

In this chapter we will discuss the effect of fibromyalgia on dental health reported in a systematic review of studies.

ORAL CAVITY SIGNS AND SYMPTOMS

Fibromyalgia has a high variation of symptoms and therefore, treatment.

A systematic review of studies in PubMed from 1997 until present day was conducted, taking into account age, gender and signs and symptoms. In a total of 9 articles, 540 patients diagnosed with fibromyalgia presented signs or symptoms in the oral cavity. The range of ages was between 38 and 71 with an average age of 50. Female patients were the most frequent, representing 91.8% of the cases. In the cases studied, the following signs and symptoms were detected, listed in order from the most frequent symptoms to the least frequent: Temporomandibular disorders (TMD): 75.20%; Xerostomia: 72.45%; Dysphagia: 37.30%; Dysgeusia: 34.20%; Glossodynia: 32.80%.

TEMPOROMANDIBULAR DISORDERS

The most common manifestations in the oral cavity are temporomandibular disorders. Patients usually also have muscle pain, trismus, arthralgia, arthritis, degenerative osteoarthritis, sounds in the jaw (clicking, popping or grating). All these manifestations are significantly more common in patients with fibromyalgia than control groups.

For the treatment of these disorders we recommend palliative therapy as well as interdisciplinary therapy, considering the psychological and systemic conditions that a patient may have.

Appointments at the dental clinic should be brief to avoid opening the mouth for a long period of time.

There are several studies about temporomandibular disorders in patients with fibromyalgia, some of them studied concrete signs and symptoms like sounds, pain in the joints and ability to open the mouth. They found significant differences among different groups, fibromyalgia being the most affected.

Other studies are based on surveys, asking about different temporomandibular disorders, with the conclusion that these disorders are more common in patients with fibromyalgia. Some studies also asked about psychological symptoms like somatization, obsessive-compulsive trends, interpersonal sensitivity, depression, anxiety, hostility, phobias, paranoid ideas and psychotic trends.

For the fibromyalgia group they found signicantly more somatization and obsessive-compulsive trends than other groups.

Xerostomia

Another common symptom is xerostomia, which may be a side effect of the medication that patients with fibromyalgia usually have to take such as antidepressants, hypnotics, muscle relaxants, painkillers and anticonvulsants. We also have to consider the psychological situation of the patient. Depression and anxiety are common.

Patients with xerostomia usually have more cervical caries, difficulty in eating, halitosis and candidiasis due to this lack of saliva.

Glossodynia

Glossodynia or burning mouth syndrome is a condition characterized by a burning or tingling sensation in the mouth.

Possible causes include anxiety, depression and hormonal disorders. Another possible cause could be hyperexcitability of the central nerve system causing hyperalgesia and allodynia (a pain due to a stimulus which does not normally provoke pain).

It is possible that one of these could be responsible for the widespread pain that patients with fibromyalgia experience.

In a clinical study about atypical pain, all patients with glossodynia were also diagnosed with fibromyalgia.

Both fibromyalgia and glossodynia are more common in women. In addition, they both have psychological consequences and both are related to hormonal disorders, hyperalgesia and sleep disorders. However, glossodynia seems to be a local disorder whereas fybromialgia has systemic affectation.

We cannot consider that burning mouth syndrome and fibromyalgia are directly related but they have some common symptoms.

Dysgeusia

Dysgeusia is the distortion of the sense of taste.

A possible cause of dysgeusia in patients with fibromyalgia could be a side effect of all the drugs that they have to take.

The drugs that are commonly used for fibromyalgia and can cause dry mouth and dysgeusia are amitriptyline, fluoxetine, venlafaxine, cyclobenzaptine and zoplicone.

MEDICAL INTERACTIONS

For all these reasons, it is important to update the clinical history frequently. We have to consider all the side effects and interactions between the drugs that the patients have to take and the drugs that we will recommend.

Tricyclic antidepressants are drugs commonly used by such patients, although there are divergent opinions.

There are some studies about interactions between amitriptyline and local anesthetics. They suggest that the use of local anesthetics with adrenaline can cause a higher risk of hypertension in patients with tricyclic antidepressant treatment.

Antibiotics of the macrolide family, namely erythromycin and clarithromycin often used in dentistry, are potent inhibitors of P-450 enzyme system, specifically the 3A4 isoform.

This enzyme is involved in the metabolization of diverse drugs usually used for the treatment of fibromyalgia, like zoplicone, venlafaxine, citalopram and zolpidem.

Consequently, the use of erythromycin and clarithromycin can cause inhibition of this enzyme and can lead to higher concentration and effect of these drugs.

CONCLUSION

It can be observed that fibromyalgia manifests itself in a number of different ways in the oral cavity, requiring a personalized therapy. We should pay special attention to TMD, relief of Xerostomia symptoms and treatment of burning mouth syndrome.

REFERENCES

Balasubramaniam R, de Leeuw R, Zhu H, Nickerson RB, Okeson JP, Carlson CR. Prevalence of temporomandibular disorders in fibromyalgia and failed back syndrome patients: a blinded prospective comparison study. *Oral Surg Oral Med Oral Pathol Oral Radiol Endod. 2007*;104:204–16.

Balasubramaniam R, Laudenbach JM, Stoopler ET. Fibromyalgia: an update for oral health care providers. *Oral Surg Oral Med Oral Pathol Oral Radiol Endod.* 2007;104:589–602.

Brown RS, Rhodus NL. Epinephrine and local anesthesia revisited. *Oral SUrg Oral Med Oral Pathol Oral Radiol Endod.* 2005;100:401–8.

Ciancio SG, editor. *ADA/PDR guide to dental therapeutics.* Chicago: American Dental Association and Thompson PDR; 2006.

Garcia Campayo J, Rodero B, Alda M, Sobradiel N, Montero J, Moreno S. Validation of the Spanish version of the Pain Catastrophizing Scale in fibromyalgia. *Med Clin (Barc).* 2008;18:131:487–92.

Giovengo SL, Russell IJ, Larson A. Increased concentrations of nerve growth factor in cerebrospinal fluid of patients with fibromyalgia. *J Reumathol.* 1999;26:1564–9.

Goulet JP, Perusse R, Turcotte JY. Contraindications to vasoconstrictors in dentistry: Part III. Pharmacologic interactions. *Oral Surg Oral Med Oral Pathol.* 1992;74:692–7.

Hedenberg-Magnusson B, Ernberg M, Kopp S. Presence of orofacial pain and temporomandibular disorder in fibromyalgia. A study by questionnaire. *Swed Dent J.* 1999;23:1948–52.

Hedenberg-Magnusson B, Ernberg M, Kopp S. Symptoms and signs of temporomandibular disorders in patients with fibromyalgia and local myalgia of the temporomandibular system: A comparative study. *Acta Odontol Scand. 1997;55:344–9.*

Hersh EV, Moore PA. Drug interactions in dentistry: the importance of knowing your CYPs. *J Am Dent Assoc.* 2004;135:298–311.

Jacobsen PL, Chavez EM. Clinical management of the dental patient taking multiple drugs. *J Contemp Dent Pract.* 2005;6:144–51.

Lavigne G, Woda A, Truclove E, Ship JA, Dao T, Goulet JP. Mechanisms associated with unusual orofacial pain. *J Orofac Pain.* 2005;19:9–21.

Leslie A, Burke M, Buchwald D. Overlapping conditions among patients with chronic fatigue syndrome, fibromyalgia and temporomandibular disorders. *Arch Inter Med.* 2000;160:221–7.

Nederfors T, Holmstro¨m G, Paulsson G, Sahlberg D. The relation between xerostomia and hyposalivation in subjects with rheumatoid arthritis or fibromyalgia. *Swed Dent J.* 2002;26:1–7.

No brega JC, Siquiera SR, Siquiera JT, Teixeira MJ. Differencial diagnosis in atypical facial pain: a clinical study. *Arq Neuropsiquiatra.* 2007;65: 256–61.

Plesh O, Wolfe F, Lane N. The relationship between fibromyalgia and temporomandibular disorders: prevalence and symptom severity. *J Reumat- hol.* 1996;23:1948–52.

Rhodus NL, Fricton J, Carlson P, Messner R. Oral symptoms associated with fibromyalgia syndrome. *J Reumathol.* 2003;30:1841–5.

Sumpton JE, Moulin DE. Fibromyalgia: presentation and management with a focus on pharmacological treatment. *Pain Res Manag.* 2008;13: 477–83.

Van Houdenhove B, Luyten P. Customizing treatment of chronic fatigue syndrome and fibromyalgia: the role of perpetuating factors. *Psychosom.* 2008;49:470–7.

Velly A, Look J, Schiffman E, Lenton P, Kang W, Messner R, Holcroft C, Fricton J. The effect of fibromyalgia and widespread pain on the clinically significant temporomandibular muscle and joint pain disorders – a prospective 18 month cohort study. *The Journal of Pain* 2010;11:1155-1164.

Wynn RL, Meiller TF, Crossley HL, editores. *Drug information handbook for dentistry* K. Hudson: Lexi-comp; 2006.

Yagiela JA. Adverse drug interactions in dental practice: interactions associated with vasoconstrictors. Part V of a serie. *J Am Dent Assoc.* 1999;130:701–9.

In: Fibromyalgia
Editor: Antonio G. Tristano
ISBN: 978-1-62257-678-4
© 2013 Nova Science Publishers, Inc.

Chapter 4

COMPLEMENTARY MEDICATIONS IN THE TREATMENT OF FIBROMYALGIA

Mario D. Cordero

Centro Andaluz de Biología del Desarrollo (CABD-CSIC),
Universidad Pablo de Olavide and Centro de Investigación
Biomédica en Red de Enfermedades Raras (CIBERER),
ISCIII, Sevilla, Spain

ABSTRACT

Fibromyalgia (FM) is a common chronic pain syndrome accompanied by other symptoms such as fatigue, headache, sleep disturbances, and depression. Pathophysiological mechanisms of FM are difficult to identify and current drug therapies demonstrate limited effectiveness, only focused to the management of single symptoms. In general, about half of all treated patients seem to experience a 30% reduction of symptoms, suggesting that many patients with FM will require additional therapies. But, in most cases, high incidence of secondary effects is induced by pharmacological therapy. In recent years, a number of innovative nutritional strategies have been proposed as safe alternative treatments to reduce the morbidity as well as the cost of treating FM. Of these, complementary supplements such as L-carnitine, D-ribose, Coenzyme Q_{10}, magnesium, S- adenosylmethionine, vitamins, etc, have been studied most extensively. However, more clinical trials are needed to determine the dose and duration of such treatments to make specific recommendations for populations with FM.

INTRODUCTION

Fibromyalgia (FM) is a common pain syndrome accompanied by other symptoms such as tender spots, decreased pain threshold, fatigue, headache, sleep disturbances, and depression. It is a chronic condition characterized by a pattern of vague symptoms that are difficult to diagnose and treat. FM is diagnosed according to the classification criteria established by the American College of Rheumatology (ACR) [1] and routine laboratory investigations usually yield normal results [2]. The prevalence of FM in industrialized countries ranges from 0,4% to 4% (it affects at least 5 million individuals in the United States and 800.000 in Spain) in the population being 11 times more frequent in women than in men [3]. Its high prevalence makes FM a major problem in developed countries in the recent years. FM causes work absenteeism and has been associated with high medical services utilization cost and considerable disability. Furthermore, the use of medications and medical necessities increased markedly across many measures once diagnosis was made. It has been estimated that annual health service cost of FM patients was twice that of patients with chronic widespread pain and pain-free controls. The fact that its diagnostic criteria are only clinical, and that its etiopathogenesis has not yet been clarified, makes the study and therapeutical approach of the disease to be very difficult. Although the etiology of FM remains unclear, evidence suggests that biological, genetic, and environmental factors are involved. It is considered that the changes in the neuronal activity in the central nervous system, abnormal metabolism of biogenic amines, immunological disorders and oxidative stress may among others factors contribute to the development of the disease. For all these reasons, it is urgent to do more research in the diagnosis, pathophysiology and therapy of FM.

FM syndrome has been related to disturbances of hypothalamic–pituitary axis together with neurotransmission imbalance, involving excitatory amino acids, catecholamines, substance P and serotonin (5-HT) [4,5,6]. Patient's symptoms may derive from poor stressor modulation, sensitization of specific nociceptor neurons and pain threshold diminution in response to multiple environmental factors, such as mechanical or emotional trauma, chronic stress or even infections. In recent years, new information to our understanding of FM pathophysiology has emerged. Some genetic polymorphisms and antibodies have been associated with FM, as the serotoninergic system genotype of 5–HTT [7,8], catechol-O-methyltransferase gene polymorphism [9], D4 dopamine receptor exon II repeat polymorphism [10], and antibodies against serotonin [11,12]. Alterations in the metabolism, transport and reuptake of serotonin [13,14] and substance P [15] have also been postulated. Moreover, cytokines homeostasis has been considered to play a role in the pathogenesis of FM [16,17]. Conversely, several studies have shown mitochondrial dysfunction and high levels of oxidative stress markers in FM patients, suggesting that this process may contribute to the pathophysiology of this disease.

THERAPEUTIC OPTIONS IN FM

The treatment of fibromyalgia is multidisciplinary, with emphasis on active patient participation, medications, cognitive-behavioral therapy and physical modalities. No single medication has yet been found that sufficiently controls all the symptoms of FM; currently available medication types include antidepressants, non-steroidal anti-inflammatory drugs, opioids, sedatives, muscle relaxants, analgesics, hypnotic agents and anticonvulsants. Clinicians can choose from a variety of pharmacological and non-pharmacological modalities. These treatments are currently focused on patient symptomatology, with deeper focus on symptoms of pain, inflammation, sleep disturbance and fatigue. We must also take into account that it is difficult to perform more or less objective valuations within the context of a fluctuating pathology like fibromyalgia.

The pharmacological treatment is currently composed of 5 groups:

a) *Antidepressants:*

Within this group of drugs, we highlight the tricyclic antidepressants, which cytotoxic effects have already been proven, [18]. Other groups of antidepressants used are MAOIs and SSRIs, which have also been demonstrated to have cytotoxic effects, [19] being these cytotoxic effects the major cause for the strong secondary effects, despite in some cases, like tricyclic antidepressants, only 40% of the subjects show recovery, [20].

b) *Anti-inflammatory:*

Numerous studies on these drugs have failed at confirming their analgesic effectiveness, [21], as well as their cytotoxic effects, [22].

c) *Antiepileptic:*

This type of drugs seem to respond adequately at treating sleep disturbances, fatigue and pain in patients with FM, but also toxic effects have been described for them, [23,24].

d) *Sedatives and muscle relaxants:*

Sedatives have been described to be effective at treating sleep disturbances and fatigue, but have poorly significant effects on pain, [25]. As for muscle relaxants, some of them, like Cyclobenzaprine, show to be highly toxic, [26,27].

e) *Opiates:*

The main problem of the treatment with this group of drugs is the secondary effects shown in the long-term, [28].

The difference between results and the secondary and cytotoxic effects of conventional treatments raise the need for the development of new drugs that improve the therapeutic efficacy and reduce the secondary and cytotoxic effects.

There are some drugs that have been proven to be efficient in pathologies like mitochondrial diseases, which show muscle disorders similar to those of FM. Furthermore, both pathologies are associated in some cases, [29,30,31]. Thereby, it is necessary to assess the therapeutic potential of some of these drugs in the treatment of FM.

COMPLEMENTARY SUPPLEMENTS

Nutritional therapy and phytotherapy have emerged as new concepts and healing systems have quickly and widely spread in recent years. Strong recommendations for consumption of nutraceuticals, natural plant foods, and the use of nutritional therapy and phytotherapy have become progressively popular to improve health, and to prevent and treat diseases. In the USA, supplements represent a market of over $7billion/year [32] and exceed $30 billion worldwide [33]. This is why the pharmaceutical industry is becoming more interested in this type of therapies.

Several nutritional and complementary elements have been studied in FM, mostly due to the knowledge on a probable deficiency in patients with FM. These treatments may be classified into different families according to their main action.

Antioxidant Treatments

In general, oxidative stress could be defined as an imbalance between the presence of high levels of ROS and reactive nitrogen species (RNS), and the antioxidative defense mechanisms. These toxic molecules are formed via oxidation-reduction reactions and are highly reactive since they have an odd number of electrons. ROS generated under physiological conditions are essential for life, as they are involved in bactericidal activity of phagocytes, and in signal transduction pathways, regulating cell growth and reduction–oxidation (redox) status [34]. ROS include free radicals, such as hydroxyl and superoxide radicals, and non-radicals, including hydrogen peroxide and singlet oxygen.

Under standard conditions, mitochondria are the main source of free radicals, but this production is controlled by antioxidants produced by the cell, such as Coenzyme Q_{10}, Vitamin E or Vitamin C; however, when this production is unbalanced with respect to that of antioxidants, numerous harmful effects appear, damaging lipids, proteins and nucleic acids.

In recent years, several studies have shown increased levels of oxidative stress markers in FM suggesting that this process may have a role in the pathophysiology of this disease. High levels of LP and protein carbonyls are two of the most documented oxidative damage markers to be associated with FM. Thus, high levels of MDA, a final product of LP, and increased levels of protein carbonyls, as a result of protein oxidation have been reported in plasma from FM patients [35,36]. Furthermore, it has been observed that total antioxidant capacity and superoxide dismutase (SOD), catalase and glutathione levels are reduced in FM patients [37,38,39].

Beneficial effects of CoQ administration in FM patients have been observed in a previous pilot study [40]. In this study, Lister et al reported beneficial effects of oral CoQ and *Gingko biloba* supplementation in FM patients. They observed an important improvement in quality-of-life scores that justified the need for a larger scale clinical trial and further investigations into the possible mechanism of action of CoQ. In our studies, oral CoQ treatment significantly improved clinical symptoms and decreased oxidative stress in several cases of FM [41,42]. Nevertheless, more controlled clinical trials are needed to provide data on the effectiveness of CoQ in FM.

Another antioxidant treatment has been assayed in FM. Melatonin, the pineal hormone with pleiotropic activity is a known powerful antioxidant and anti-inflammatory and increasing experimental and clinical evidence show its beneficial effects against oxidative/nitrosative stress status, including that involving mitochondrial dysfunction [43]. Treatment of FM patients with 3 mg melatonin daily for 30 days significantly improved the tender point count, severity of pain, global physical assessments, and sleep [44]. Moreover, in a limited number of cases, administration of 6 mg/day melatonin to patients with FMS resulted in normal sleep/wake cycles, normal diurnal activity, lack of pain, and fatigue and claims significant improvement of the behavioral symptoms including lack of depression [45]. Recently, in a double-blind, placebo-controlled clinical study was demonstrated that administration of melatonin, alone or in a combination with fluoxetine, was effective in the treatment of patients with FM [46]. The "Myers' cocktail", an intravenous vitamin-and-mineral formula (IVMT) for the treatment of a wide range of clinical conditions, which has vitamin C as an antioxidant, has also been assayed also, and most subjects experienced relief as compared to baseline, but no statistically significant differences were seen between IVMT and placebo [47].

Vitamin D, which controls calcium and phosphorus metabolism [48], is also a membrane antioxidant [49] whose deficiency has been linked to chronic pain, muscle weakness [50,51] and FM [52]. Subsequently, studies evaluating the effects of high-dose vitamin D treatment have been demonstrated to improve clinical symptoms in FM [53].

Treatment Based on Mitochondrial Function

Mitochondria are dynamic organelles that play a central role in many cellular functions including the generation of chemical energy (adenosine triphosphate, ATP), heat, and intracellular calcium homeostasis. They are also responsible for the formation of reactive oxygen species (ROS) and for triggering the programmed cell death or apoptosis [54]. The primary metabolic function of mitochondria is oxidative phosphorylation, an energy-generating process that couples oxidation of respiratory substrates to the synthesis of ATP. The mitochondrial respiratory chain (MRC) is composed of five multisubunit enzyme complexes; Complex I (NADH:ubiquinone oxidoreductase); II (Succinate dehydrogenase); III (cytochrome bc1 complex); IV (cytochrome c oxidase); V (F_OF_1 ATP synthase complex). Both mitochondrial DNA (mtDNA) and nuclear DNA (nDNA) encode for polypeptide components of these complexes. Electron transport between MRC complexes I–IV is coupled to the extrusion of protons across the inner mitochondrial membrane by proton pump components of the respiratory chain.

This movement of protons creates an electrochemical gradient ($\Delta\Psi$m) across the inner mitochondrial membrane. Protons return to the mitochondrial matrix by flowing through ATP synthase (complex V), which utilizes the energy thus produced to synthesize ATP from adenosine diphosphate (ADP) and inorganic phosphate (Pi). Both mtDNA and nDNA encode for polypeptide components of these complexes. As a consequence, mutations in either genome can cause MRC dysfunctions that impair transport of electron and/or proton transport and decrease ATP synthesis. Primary or secondary genetic diseases affecting MRC or secondary mitochondrial dysfunctions usually affect brain tissues and skeletal muscle because of their energy requirements. Besides MRC enzyme complexes, two electron carriers, CoQ_{10} and cytochrome c, are essential for mitochondrial synthesis of ATP. CoQ transports electrons from complexes I and II to complex III and is essential for the stability of complex III. CoQ is a lipid-soluble component of virtually all cell membranes. It is composed of a benzoquinone ring with a polyprenyl side-chain. The number of isoprene units is specie specific, e.g. 10 in humans (CoQ10). CoQ also functions as an antioxidant that protects cells both by direct ROS scavenging and by regenerating other antioxidants such as vitamins C and E [55].

One of these important functions that could be necessary to improve is the mitochondrial respiratory chain, by either providing electrons to the complexes of this chain for their adequate functioning or by trying to improve the activity of those complexes that function inadequately.

- *Coenzyme Q_{10}:* It acts accepting and transferring electrons from Complexes I and II to Complex III of the respiratory chain. Furthermore, it is a powerful antioxidant, and its effectiveness has been proven in different pathologies [56], and with satisfactory results in FM, although in non-controlled assays [40,41,42].
- *Ibedenone:* This drug has a structure and function similar to those of coenzyme Q, but it is more soluble and capable of crossing the blood-brain barrier. It has been tested in pathologies like MELAS [57] which, as previously mentioned, has been already related to FM [29]; therefore, it could be considered as a new option in the treatment of FM.
- *Tiamine o Vitamin B1:* It acts as a cofactor of pyruvate dehydrogenase, which is a mitochondrial enzyme that transforms piruvate into acetyl-CoA for the Krebs cycle, thus stimulating the respiratory chain. It has been related already to FM regarding concentration and treatment alterations, [58].

- *Creatine monohydrate:* Creatine is synthesized in our organism acting as energy storage of phosphate groups for the phosphorylation of ADP to ATP, and it has a week antioxidant potential. In the case of FM, some case has already been described about deficiency and treatment with creatine with satisfactory results for the patient on depressive symptoms, [59].
- *Carnitine:* It transports fatty acids inside the mitochondria to produce β-oxidation and to regulate the concentrations of free intra-mitochondrial Coenzyme A. An alteration of the mitochondrial chain may trigger a secondary alteration of β-oxidation of fatty acids, causing an accumulation of fatty acids and, therefore, carnitine deficiency. Its administration has been proven to be efficient in pathologies with mitochondrial alteration, [60]. Alterations in carnitine levels in patients with FM have been proven as well, [61]. To this respect, L-carnitine has been tested in patients with FM, showing interesting improvement in pain and mental and general health of patients [62].

Treatment of Minerals

- *Selenium and Magnesium:* Selenium, besides being a mineral, is an essential element in several metabolic pathways, including the glutathione peroxidase pathway. Selenium seems to promote antioxidant activity in the organism through glutathione peroxidase, a selenium-dependent enzyme. It has been proven that there are concentration alterations of this enzyme in FM, as it is the case of magnesium as well, which has diverse metabolic functions and plays an important role in the production and transport of energy. It is also useful in muscle contraction and relaxation, [63,64], and there are evidence on the benefits of the exogenous administration of both selenium and magnesium, [65,66], but there are few data that confirm this.

Other Treatments

- Malic Acid: Malic acid is a main component of the Krebs cycle. Its role is to participate in the complex process of adenosine triphosphate

(ATP) production. So far, there are few data that confirm its benefits in FM from a scientific point of view, [67].

- Deutrosulfazyme (Cellfood®): Cellfood is an innovative nutritional supplement containing 78 ionic/colloidal trace elements and minerals combined with 34 enzymes and 17 amino acids, all suspended in a solution of deuterium sulfate. Recently, a randomized placebo-controlled trial, Cellfood's therapy has shown to improve FM symptoms and health-related quality of life [68]. Nevertheless, more controlled clinical trials are needed to provide data on the effectiveness of Cellfood in FM.

- *D-Ribose:* Ribose is a simple carbohydrate that plays a role in high-energy phosphate and nucleic acid synthesis. Ribose bypasses the rate-limiting enzymatic steps of the pentose phosphate pathway and accelerates the formation of ATP and subsequent tissue recovery. D-ribose has shown to significantly reduce clinical symptoms in patients suffering from FM and chronic fatigue syndrome [69].

- *S-adenosylmethionine:* is a naturally occurring molecule that serves as a methyl donor in human cellular metabolism, considered as a relatively new anti-inflammatory drug with analgesic and anti-depressant effects. Oral treatment with S-adenosylmethionine has some beneficial effects on primary FM in pain, fatigue, and morning stiffness parameters [70]. However, in another study, intravenous administration, compared to placebo, showed no effect of S-adenosylmethionine in patients with FM [71].

- *Chlorella pyrenoidosa*: is a freshwater unicellular green alga which contains abundant proteins and chlorophyll compared to other plants, and also large quantities of minerals, such as iron and magnesium, and vitamins, such as folate, vitamin B-6, vitamin B-12 and essential amino acids required for human growth and health [72]. In FM, it has been used in only one study, showing decrease in pain intensity [73]; however, more comprehensive double-blind, placebo-controlled clinical trials in these patients are warranted.

FUTURE PERSPECTIVES

There are numerous therapeutic options that have shown some degree of efficiency in the treatment of the symptoms of FM. However, we are still far from finding the adequate treatment for FM; a treatment that covers the more symptoms, with the lesser degree of secondary effects for the patient. The high complexity degree of this disease requires a multidisciplinary treatment. However, it would be interesting to explore those therapeutic options that have shown deficiency in the patients. CoQ_{10} plays a crucial role in cellular metabolism acting as the electron carrier between complexes I and II and the complex III of the mitochondrial respiratory chain; and regulates uncoupling proteins, the transition pore, β-oxidation of fatty acids, and nucleotide pathway [55]. CoQ_{10} deficiency has been associated to a variety of human disorders, some of them caused by a direct defect of CoQ_{10} biosynthesis genes or as a secondary event [35]. Interestingly, patients with CoQ_{10} deficiency display improvement of symptoms, sometimes dramatic, after oral CoQ10 supplementation [74]. Tiamine, creatine and carnitine have also shown some degree of deficiency in patients with FM [58,59,61].

From another perspective, these therapeutic complements of the treatment of FM could be considered as coadjuvant or co-treatments, combined with other drugs of common use in FM. CoQ_{10} and carnitine have shown a high degree of efficiency combined with amitriptyline in the treatment of cyclic vomiting syndrome, in which a mitochondrial dysfunction has already been described [75].

Finally, normal cell function is maintained by nutrients from foods and endogenous antioxidants. Consequently, it seems reasonable to use some form of these same nutrients and antioxidants to correct cell dysfunction, a concept that is especially relevant for FM, where cells are particularly low in many nutrients and antioxidants. At the present time, nutritional and antioxidant therapies may provide more benefits, with fewer adverse consequences, than conventional medications.

REFERENCES

[1]   F. Wolfe, H.A. Smythe, M.B. Yunus, R.M. Bennett, C. Bombardier, D.L. Goldenberg, P. Tugwell, S.M. Campbell, M. Abeles, P. Clark, A.G. Fam, S.J. Farber, J.J. Fiechtner, C.M. Franklin, R.A. Gatter, D. Hamaty, J. Lessard, A.S. Lichtbroun, A.T. Masi, G.A. Mccain, W.J. Reynolds, T.J. Romano, I.J. Russell, R.P. Sheon. *Arthritis Rheum.* 33, 2, (1990).

[2]   M. Yunus, A.T. Masi, J.J. Calabro, K.A. Miller, S.L. Feigenbaum. *Semin Arthritis Rheum.* 11, 1, (1981).

[3]   R.C. Lawrence, D.T. Felson, C.G. Helmick, L.M. Arnold, H. Choi, R.A. Deyo, S. Gabriel, R. Hirsch, M.C. Hochberg, G.G. Hunder, J.M. Jordan, J.N. Katz, H.M. Kremers, F. Wolfe. *Arthritis Rheum.* 58, 1, (2008).

[4]   I.J. Russell, M.D. Orr, B. Littman, G.A. Vipraio, D. Alboukrek, J.E. Michalek, Y. Lopez, F. MacKillip. *Arthritis Rheum.* 37, 11, (1994).

[5]   L.J. Crofford, N.C. Engleberg, and M.A. Demitrack. *Baillieres Clin Rheumatol.* 10, 2, (1996).

[6]   G. Neeck. *Ageing Res Rev.* 1, 2, (2002).

[7]   L. Bazzichi, G. Giannaccini, L. Betti, P. Italiani, L. Fabbrini, F. Defeo, C. Giacomelli, T. Giuliano, A. Rossi, A. Uccelli, L. Giusti, G. Mascia, A. Lucacchini, S. Bombardieri. *Clinical Biochem.* 39, 9, (2006).

[8]   B. Tander, S. Gunes, O. Boke, G. Alayli, N. Kara, H. Bagci, and F. Canturk. *Rheumatol Int.* 28, 7, (2008).

[9]   S. Gursoy, E. Erdal, H. Herken, E. Madenci, B. Alasehirli, and N. Erdal. *Rheumatol Int.* 23, 3, (2003).

[10]   D. Buskila, H. Cohen, L. Neumann, and R.P. Ebstein. *Mol Psychiatry.* 9, 8, (2004).

[11]   R. Klein, M. Beansch, and P.A. Berg. *Psychoneuroendocrinology.* 17, 5, (1992).

[12]   E. Werle, H. Fisher, A. Muller, W. Fiehn, W. Eich. *J Rheumatol.* 28, 3, (2001).

[13]   M.N.Y. Alnigenis, and P. Barland. *Clin Exp Rheumatol* 19, 2, (2001).

[14]   M.J. Schwarz, M. Offenbaecher, A. Neumeister, T. Ewert, M. Willeit, N. Praschak-Rieder, J. Zach, M. Zacherl, K. Lossau, R. Weisser, G. Stucki, M. Ackenheil. *Neurobiol Dis.* 11, 3, (2002).

[15]   R. Staud and M. Spaeth. *CNS Spectr.* 13, 3 Suppl 5, (2008).

[16]   D.J. Wallace, M. Linker-Israeli, D. Hallegua, S. Silverman, D. Silver, and M.H. Weisman. *Rheumatology (Oxford).* 40, 7, (2001).

[17]   D.J. Wallace. *Curr Pharm Des.* 12, 1, (2006).

[18]   A.M. Moreno-Fernández, M.D. Cordero, J. Garrido-Maraver, E. Alcocer-Gómez, N. Casas-Barquero, M.I. Carmona-López, J.A. Sánchez-Alcázar, M. de Miguel. J Psychiatr Res. http://dx.doi.org/10.1016/j.jpsychires.2011.11.002.

[19]   N.D. Slamon and V.W. Pentreath. *Chem Biol Interact.* 14,127, (2000).

[20]   G.O. Littlejohn and E.K. Guymer. Curr Pharm Des. 12,1, 2006.

[21]   J. Lautenschlager. *Scand J Rheumatol.* Suppl,113, (2000).

[22]   M. Petruzzelli, A. Moschetta, W. Renooij, M.B. de Smet, G. Palasciano, P. Portincasa and K.J. van Erpecum. *Dig Dis Sci.* 51,4, (2006).

[23] I. Rodriguez-Blanco, D. Sanchez-Aguilar and J. Toribio. *Actas Dermosifiliogr.* 96,2, (2005).

[24] S.P. Varghese, L.R. Haith, M.L. Patton, R.E. Guilday and B.H. Ackerman. *Pharmacotherapy.* 26,5, (2006).

[25] J. Lautenschlager. *Scand J Rheumatol.* Suppl,113, (2000).

[26] H.A. Spiller, M.L. Winter, K.V. Mann, D.J. Borys, S. Muir and E.P. Krenzelok. *J Emerg Med.* 13,6, (1995).

[27] S.B. Chabria. J Occup Med Toxicol. 17,1, (2006).

[28] R.M. Bennett. *South Med J.* 97,5, (2004).

[29] R.A. DeSouza, R.J. Cardenas, T.U. Lindler, F.A. De la Fuente, F.J. Mayorquin, D.S. Trochtenberg. *South Med J.* 97,5, (2004).

[30] J. Benito-León, A. Berbel, J. Porta-Estessam, A. Martínez, J. Arenas. *Rev Neurol.* 24,134, (1996).

[31] M. Villanova, E. Selvi, A. Malandrini, C. Casali, F.M. Santorelli, R. De Stefano, R. Marcolongo. *Muscle Nerve.* 22,2, (1999).

[32] V. Glaser. *Nature Biotechnology.* 17,1, (1999).

[33] I. Raskin, D. M. Ribnicky, S. Komarnytsky, N. Ilic, A. Poulev, N. Borisjuk, A. Brinker, D.A. Moreno, C. Ripoll, N. Yakoby, J.M. O'Neal, T. Cornwell, I. Pastor, B. Fridlender. *Trends in Biotechnology.* 20,12, (2002).

[34] K.J. Davies. *Biochem Soc Symp.* 61,1–31, (1995).

[35] M.D. Cordero, A.M. Moreno-Fernández, M. deMiguel, P. Bonal, F. Campa, L.M. Jiménez-Jiménez, A. Ruiz-Losada, B. Sánchez-Domínguez, J.A. Sánchez Alcázar, L. Salviati, P. Navas. *Clin Biochem.* 42,7-8, (2009).

[36] O. Altindag, A. Gur, N. Calgan, N. Soran, H. Celik, and S. Selek. *Redox Rep.* 12,3, (2007).

[37] O. Altindag and H Celik. *Redox Rep.* 11,3, (2006).

[38] S. Bagis, L. Tamer, G. Sahin, R. Bilgin, H. Guler, B. Ercan, C. Erdogan. *Rheumatol Int.* 25,3, (2005).

[39] O.F. Sendur, Y. Turan, E. Tastaban, C. Yenisey, M. Serter. *Rheumatol Int.* 29,6, (2009).

[40] R.E. Lister. J Int Med Res. 30,2, (2002)

[41] M.D. Cordero, E. Alcocer-Gómez, F.J. Cano-García, M. de Miguel, F. Campa, P. Bona, A.M. Moreno Fernández. *J Muscoskel Pain.* 19, 2, (2011).

[42] M.D. Cordero, E. Alcocer-Gómez, M. de Miguel, F.J. Cano-García, C.M. Luque, P. Fernández-Riejo, A.M. Fernández, J.A. Sánchez-Alcazar. *Mitochondrion.* 11, 4, (2011).

[43] D. Acuña-Castroviejo, L.C. López, G. Escames, A. López, J.A. García, R.J. Reiter. *Curr Top Med Chem.* 11, 2, (2011).

[44] G. Citera, A. Arias, J.A. Maldonado-Cocco, M.A. Lázaro, M.G. Rosemffet, L.I. Brusco, E.J. Scheines, D.P. Cardinalli. *Clin Rheumatol.* 19, 1, (2000).

[45] D. Acuna-Castroviejo, G. Escames, R.J. Reiter RJ. *J Pineal Res,* 40,1, (2006).

[46] S.A. Hussain, I.I. Al-Khalifa, N.A. Jasim, F.I. Gorial. *J Pineal Res.* 50, 3, (2011).

[47] A. Ali, V.Y. Njike, V. Northrup, A.B. Sabina, A.L. Williams, L.S. Liberti, A.I. Perlman, H. Adelson, D.L. Katz. *J Altern Complement Med.* 15, 3, (2009).

[48] A.W. Norman, I. Nemere, L.X. Zhou, J.E. Bishop, K.E. Lowe, A.C. Maiyar, E.D. Collins, T. Taoka, I. Sergeev, M.C. Farach-Carson. *J Steroid Biochem Mol Biol.* 41,3-8, (1992).

[49] H. Wiseman. FEBS Lett. 326, 1-3, (1993).

[50] S. Straube, R. Andrew Moore, S. Derry, H.J. McQuay. *PAIN.* 141, 1-2, (2009).

[51] R. Zhang, D.P. Naughton. *Nutr J.* 8, 9, (2010).

[52] D.J. Armstrong, G.K.; Meenagh, I. Bickle, A.S. Lee, E.S. Curran, M.B. Finch. *Clin Rheumatol.* 26, 4, (2007).

[53] H. Badsha, M. Daher, K.O. Kong. *Clin Rheumatol.* 28, 8, (2009).

[54] J.F. Turrens. *J Physiol.* 552,2, (2003).

[55] M. Turunen, J. Olsson, G. Dallner. *Biochim Biophys Acta.* 1660, 1-2, (2004).

[56] M. Dhanasekaran and J. Ren. *Curr Neurovasc Res.* 2,5, (2005).

[57] Y. Ihara, R. Namba, S. Kuroda, T. Sato, T. Shirabe. *J Neurol Sci.* 90,3, (1989).

[58] J. Eisinger. J Am Coll Nutr. 17,3, (1998).

[59] D. Amital, T. Vishne, A. Rubinow, J. Levine. *Am J Psychiatry.* 163,10, (2006).

[60] S. DiMauro, M. Mancuso, A. Naini. *Ann N.Y. Sci.* 1011, (2004).

[61] A. Bengtsson, G. Cederblad, J. Larsson. *Clin Exp Rheumatol.* 8,2, (1990).

[62] M. Rossini, O. Di Munno, G. Valentini, G. Bianchi, G. Biasi, E. Cacace, D. Malesci, G. La Montagna, O. Viapiana, S. Adami. *Clin Exp Rheumatol.* 25,2, (2007).

[63] J. Eisinger, A. Plantamura, P.A. Marie, T. Ayavou. Magnes Res. 7,3-4, (1994).

[64]   M. Magaldi, L. Moltoni, G. Biasi, R. Marcolongo. *Minerva Med.* 91,7-8, (2000).

[65]   D.E. Moulin. *Clin J Pain.* 17,4, (2001).

[66]   M.F. Robinson, D.R. Campbell, R.D. Stewart, H.M. Rea, C.D. Thomson, P.G. Snow, I.H. Squires. *N Z Med J.* 13,93, (1981).

[67]   I.J. Russell, J.E. Michalek, J.D. Flechas, G.E. Abraham. *J Rheumatol.* 22,5, (1995).

[68]   M.E. Nieddu, L. Menza, F. Baldi, B. Frediani, R. Marcolongo. *Reumatismo.* 59,4, (2007).

[69]   J.E. Teitelbaum, C. Johnson, J. St Cyr. *J Altern Complement Med.* 12,9, (2006).

[70]   S. Jacobsen, B. Danneskiold-Samsøe, R.B. Andersen. *Scand J Rheumatol.* 20,4, (1991).

[71]   H. Volkmann, J. Nørregaard, S. Jacobsen, B. Danneskiold-Samsøe, G. Knoke, D. Nehrdich. *Scand J Rheumatol.* 26,3, (1997).

[72]   R.E. Merchant, C.A. Andre. *Altern Ther Health Med.*7,3, (2001).

[73]   R.E. Merchant, C.A. Carmack, C.M. Wise. *Phytother Res.* 14,3, (2000).

[74]   G. Montini, C. Malaventura, L. Salviati. N. *Engl. J. Med.* 358, (2008).

[75]   R.G. Boles. *BMC Neurol.* 16,11, (2011).

In: Fibromyalgia   ISBN: 978-1-62257-678-4
Editor: Antonio G. Tristano   © 2013 Nova Science Publishers, Inc.

Chapter 5

FIBROMYALGIA: THE ROLE OF ANTIDEPRESSANT AGENTS

**M. D. Schafranski, A. B. Merlini, A. L. O. Prestes,
B. Ribeiro, J. G. Silva and M. F. Gauer**
Faculty of Medicine Universidade Estadual de Ponta Grossa (UEPG),
State of Parana, Brazil

1. INTRODUCTION

Fibromyalgia (FM) is a prevalent, chronic and disabling disorder, which etiology is unknown. It is characterized by widespread pain, diffuse tenderness, and a plethora of other symptoms. It is also considered the coexistence of tender points – painful points when a digital palpation of 4 kg/A of force is exercised - through the body. [1]

Technically, it can be defined as a history of widespread pain for at least 3 months and the existence of pain at least in 11 of 18 tender points. [2]

Its manifestations are not homogenous, making the diagnosis difficult. It shows varying proportions of anxiety and depression as comorbidities, which depend on the psychological features of each patient. Therefore, the medical evaluation must not include only the presence/absence of widespread pain or painful tender points, but also the existence of mood changes. [3]

Some studies show that the patients with FM have high rates of alexithymia and rage, and link depression, work stress and childhood traumatic events as contributors to its etiology, therefore, antidepressants could be an effective therapeutic handling. [3,4]

On the other hand, researchers have identified the influence of social effort and emotional context under the pain threshold in FM. These and other results led to conclude that there is an intrinsic bind between depressive disorders and FM. Other studiers classified them in a same wide category of stress disturbances. [4]

Finally, depression is a frequent (present in 28,6 to 70% of the patients) comorbidity associated with fibromyalgia, and brings worsening to its natural history of disease. [5]

2. HISTORY

Unfortunately, until a few decades ago, fibromyalgia was considered by many physicians and researchers as a psychological condition. During the 20 [th] century, it was finally classified as a real physical disorder. [6]

At the beginning of studies, in view of the main symptom − muscle pain, the presence of damage in fibrous and muscular tissues was considered. However, with the advance of histopathological exams, this damage was not observed. [7]

The existence of autoimmune processes in its pathophysiology was also contemplated, but no immune system disorders − which explain them - were found. [7,8]

Eventually, on the 21th century, with the rise of modern laboratory methods and brain-imaging techniques, researchers have identified a model of sensitization in central nervous system in patients with FM. Today ongoing researches continue to uncover exciting new information involving the causes and treatment of this syndrome. Consequently, an abridge timeline shows the main discoveries in the study of FM. [8]

3. EPIDEMIOLOGY

According to epidemiological studies, FM affects 5 million Americans with 18 years old or more, being 80-90% composed by women. The majority of diagnosis is established in middle age, but its symptoms can appear earlier. [9]

Table 1. Timeline of major events in the study of fibromyalgia [6,7,8]

Period	Researcher	Description
Ancient Medicine	Hippocrates	Plaques of bigger consistency in muscles of rheumatoid patients
1842	Robert Friedrich Frorie	The plaques were named "muscular calluses"
1904	William Gowers Ralph Stockman	The term "fibrositis" was created to describe the presence of fibrous tissue inflammation in rheumatoid muscles. It was reported the existence of extremely sensitiveness to pressure nodes in patients with FM. The biopsy revealed inflammatory hyperplasia in these areas.
1912	Arthur Basset Jones *et al.*	A monograph highlighted the presence of rheumatoid muscles and fibrositis.
1970's	Harvey Moldovsky Yunus *et al.*	Described the presence of sleep disturbs, as well as the role of neurotransmitters (serotonin and substance P) in its pathophysiology. Reported the concomitance of somatic syndromes: irritable bowel, headaches; as well as psychiatric disturbances: irritability, anxiety, hypochondria and even hysteria.
1976	Philip Kahler Hench	In view of the inexistence of specific inflammatory proof, the term "fibrositis" was replaced by "fibromyalgia".
1981	Muhammad B. Yunus and Alphonse T. Mais	Achievement of the first controlled trial, which brought the validation of known symptoms and tender points. The term "fibromyalgia" became universally accepted.
1987	American Medical Association	Recognized fibromyalgia as a real physical condition.

Table 1. (Continued)

Period	Researcher	Description
1990	American College of Rheumatology	Developed the diagnostic criteria to be used by physicians; the participation of neurohormonal mechanism with central sensitization was established.
2007	Food and Drug Administration	Approval of the first drug for the treatment of fibromyalgia.

The prevalence in general population is about 2%, but it booms with the age, being higher in women on fifth to seventh decades (7.4-10%). [10]

Recent studies indicate FM as the third most common rheumatic disease, behind osteoarthritis and lumbago. In Europe, the prevalence was 4,7% for chronic widespread pain, and 2,9% for strong pain and fatigue. [11]

The distribution of the disease by sex does not change in children. 15% of cases seen in rheumatologic clinics are attributed to FM, and 6% in other specialties, showing the incredible increase of its incidence. [12]

3.1. RISK FACTORS

Due to multifactorial features that compose FM, the determination of its risk factors became an arduous study. [13]

Some researchers associate its development to physical or emotional stressful or traumatic events. Others believe in the succession of repetitive injuries, bind to another disease, or believe that it occurs spontaneously. [14]

Several studies involve the processing pain made by the central nervous system (CNS), and the regulator role of genes in detecting the painful stimuli. [13]

In the presence of a positive family history, the chances of developing FM are increased, having the heredity and environmental factors as possible responsibles. [14]

Wolf *et al.* gathered some events as risk factors:

Table 2. Main described risk factors [3,13,14]

Risk Factors
Depression (hospitalization, present or current treatment, familiar historic)
Elevated levels of somatization and anxiety
Articular stroke sensation
Paresthesia and morning rigidity
Sleep disorders
Irritable bowel
Bad perception or satisfaction of health state
Traumatic events
Febrile diseases
Gender (> 7x in women)
Age (more frequent on the 5th to the 7th decades)
Family history

4. CLINICAL MANIFESTATIONS

Fibromyalgia (FM) was diagnosed based on the ARC 1990 criteria until recently [15], which was the evaluation of the widespread pain in combination with tenderness at 11 or more of 18 specific tender point sites. Lately, the provisional ARC 2010 fibromyalgia diagnostic criteria [16] proposed an alternative method to diagnose FM, this one does not require the presence of tenderness, but rather includes a list of several other symptoms: fatigue, unrefreshing sleep, and cognitive symptoms are the most important. There is still a mix of some other symptoms that might include headache, depression, and lower abdominal pain or cramping. [17] The hallmark symptom is surely the widespread pain.

The diagnosis of FM requires these symptoms. Nevertheless, a patient must also have some of the other symptoms that are common among FM patients in order to reach a composite score that would lead to a diagnosis of FM. Some experimental studies have identified a number of other abnormalities in FM patients, including increased sensitivity to multiple types of painful stimuli, increased sensitivity to other sensory modalities, and alterations in pain modulator mechanisms. [17] The quality of life in FM patients can be significantly compromised, as it can interfere with a patient's ability to work and perform regular daily activities.

Table 3. Main symptoms of fibromyalgia

Symptom	Description
Sleep Disturbances	Poor sleep occurs in about 70% to 75% of fibromyalgia patients. Morning fatigue, which is a clearer indicator of nonrestorative sleep, is present in about 75% to 80% of fibromyalgia patients. Nonrestorative sleep, or waking feeling unrefreshed, are common complaints among fibromyalgia patients. [18]
Fatigue	Fatigue occurs in 80% to 90% of fibromyalgia patients and is generally characterized by exhaustion, lack of energy, and a feeling of generalized weakness. Fatigue or exhaustion is sometimes more difficult for some patients to deal with than widespread pain. [18]
Headache	Tension type headaches and migraines are present in more than 50% of patients with fibromyalgia. Migraine is associated with an enhanced response and hyperalgesia to various stimuli such as mechanical pressure, heat, cold, sound, and light. [18] Central sensitization may be a common pathway for headaches in fibromyalgia patients considering the high prevalence of headaches in fibromyalgia [19]
Psychiatric disorders	Many studies have indicated that fibromyalgia is strongly associated with depressive and anxiety symptoms, as well as personal and family history of depression and accompanying antidepressant treatment. [20] Fibromyalgia is associated with a significantly higher rate of mood and anxiety disorders and more somatic symptoms compared to patients that have other chronic pain conditions, such as rheumatoid arthritis. [21]

5. PATHOPHYSIOLOGY

Investigators have come to agree that the pathophysiology of fibromyalgia is due to abnormal central pain mechanisms. However, there seems to be a number of central nervous system processes in the brain and in the spinal cord that have documented abnormalities in patients with fibromyalgia. [22]

5.1. Altered Pain Perception in FM Patients

Subjective measurements of pain, objective evaluations of peripheral pain reflexes, and brain imaging studies have indicated that patients with fibromyalgia experience pain differently from healthy individuals. FM patients have physiologically lower pain thresholds. There are also differences in pain processing. The threshold in which normal stimuli (pressure, heat, and cold) becomes painful is lower in patients with fibromyalgia. In fact, many evidences indicate that tender points are just sites normally more sensitive to pressure pain in all individuals [17] and that FM patients have increased pressure sensitivity at non-tender-point sites as well. There are some studies which show that FM patients have increased sensitivity to many kinds of painful stimulation, including pressure on non-tender-point sites, [23] heat and cold pain, [24,25] electrical stimulation, [24] and intramuscular hypertonic saline injection. [26]

5.2. Central Sensization

Central sensitization is an enhanced excitability of the spinal cord neurons that transmit pain information to the brain through C-fibers. Central sensitization seems to be the main contributing factor for the hyperalgesia that is experienced in fibromyalgia. Central sensitization is associated with spontaneous nerve activity, expanded receptive fields, and augmented stimulus responses within the spinal cord. Abnormal temporal summation ("wind-up") is the phenomenon whereby after an initial painful stimulus subsequent equal stimuli are perceived to be more intensely painful. This magnified "second pain," which occurs in everyone, is exaggerated in patients with fibromyalgia. [27]

These enhanced responses could be related to one or more of several possible factors: (1) an ongoing peripheral source of input from C-nociceptors other than the applied stimulus; (2) sensitized Nmethyl- D-aspartic acid (NMDA) receptors in central nociceptive neurons; (3) abnormalities in descending modulation; (4) abnormal processing at supraspinal levels. [17]

Despite the fact that the specific abnormalities leading to enhanced excitability of these neurons is not known, increasing evidence indicates that patients with FB experience abnormal pain amplification at the level of the spine.

5.3. Neurotransmitters

Serotonin is a neurotransmitter produced by neurons in the brainstem and derived from tryptophan. Serotonin has some inhibitory effects on several pain pathways and is widely distributed. Increased serotonin in the brain leads to blunted pain signaling via decreased release of P substance in the spinal cord. [22]

6. DIAGNOSIS

In spite of the advance of diagnostic medicine, the identification of FM covers 75% of affected patients, and when it is made, lasts an average of 5 years. [4]

As in other disorders, complete anamnesis and physical examination is required to establish the diagnostic, being the laboratory and radiologic exams necessary only in the presence of comorbities, or to move away other possibilities. [4]

When evaluating the joints, the presence of swelling, tenderness (allodynia/hyperalgesia), crepitus or motion alterations must be reported, as well as weakness or abnormal pain peripheral generation. [4]

The history of widespread pain for at least 3 months and the existence of pain at least in 11 of 18 tender points, as explained previously, was defined for the first time by the American College of Rheumatology, in 1990, as the diagnostic criteria for FM.2 [28]

The conception of tender point follows the Manual Tender Point Survey (MTPS) method, a classification which increased the sensibility and specificity of its diagnosis, based on:

a. Location
b. Patient and examiner positioning
c. Pressure technique
d. Severity rating scores: 0 (absence of pain) – 10 (unbearable pain); a score of 2 points characterizes a tender point as positive [29]

Aftermost, Wolf *et al.* created a new model of diagnostic criteria, which does not involve the presence of tender points, but the existence of somatic symptoms. [30]

7. GENETIC CONSIDERATIONS

In view of the presence of several cases in a same family, the role of genes in the pathophysiology of FM is being discussed for decades. [31]

However, the studies have not demonstrated concrete results yet. There are evidences appointing to non-specific polymorphisms on serotoninergic, catecholaminergic and dopaminergic circuits linked to their etiopathogenesis. [32]

8. TREATMENT

8.1. Non-pharmacological Treatment

A multidisciplinary therapy is a key issue in fibromyalgia. The treatment of fibromyalgia is a set of pharmacological treatment, change of lifestyle and non-pharmacological treatment. It is the role of the physician to establish a good relationship with the patient. The medical professional must also encourage the patient the change of lifestyle and non-pharmacological treatment defending its effectiveness. The measures include early treatment of infections, aerobic or anaerobic exercise as prescribed by the doctor, stretching, healthy sleep, avoid mood swings, treatment of depression and anxiety, group therapy, and if necessary, psychiatric counseling, among others. [33,34]

Table 4. Analgesics used in FM treatment

Analgesics				
	Mechanism of Action	**Metabolism**	**Excretion**	**Common side effects**
Tramadol [36,38,40]	It binds to upload receptors in the CNS, inhibits ascending pain pathways; also inhibits norepinephrine and serotonin reuptake	Hepatic metabolism	Urine	Flushing, itching, constipation, nausea, weakness, dizziness, headache, drowsiness, insomnia

There are several studies indicating the benefits of a plethora of non-pharmacological management of FM, such as: hydrotherapy, physiotherapy, acupuncture, cognitive-behavioral therapy, and others, some of them indicated as adjuvant, improving the patients' quality of life [35]

Table 5. Antidepressants used for FM management

Antidepressants				
	Mechanism of Action	**Metabolism**	**Excretion**	**Common side effects**
Amitriptyline [36,37,38,40,41,43,45]	It increases the synaptic concentration of serotonin in and norepinephrine in the CNS by inhibition of reuptake of them	Hepatic metabolism by CYP450, 2C19, 1A2 and 2D6.	Urine and faeces	Blurred vision, constipation, diarrhea, dizziness, dry mouth, headache, loss of appetite, nausea, trouble sleeping, weakness
Duloxetine [36,38,39]	It Inhibits the neuronal reuptake of serotonin and norepinephrine and weak inhibitor of dopamine uptake	Hepatic metabolism by CYP1A2 and 2D6	Urine and faeces	Nausea, dry mouth, headache, constipation, trouble sleeping
Milnacipran [36,38,39,41]	It inhibits the reuptake of norepinephrine and serotonin, especially the first one.	Conjugation	Urine	Nausea, headache, constipation, insomnia
Venlafaxine [36,40]	It inhibits the neuronal reuptake of serotonin and norepinephrine and weak inhibitor of dopamine uptake.	Hepatic metabolism by CYP2D6	Urine	Headache, nausea, insomnia, asthenia, dizziness, ejaculation disorder, somnolence, dry mouth, sweating
Desvenlafaxine [36,40]	It inhibits the neuronal reuptake of serotonin and norepinephrine.	Conjugation	Urine	Nausea, headache, dizziness, dry mouth, hyperhidrosis, diarrhea, constipation

8.2. Pharmacotherapy

Pharmacologic therapy of fibromyalgia includes antidepressants (they decrease pain and improve patient's quality of life), analgesics (they act reducing pain and improving the patient's quality of life), anxiolytics (useful in the management of anxiety and improves sleep quality), muscle relaxants (they relieve muscle tension and chronic pain), anticonvulsants (management of chronic pain, depressed patients and patients who report sleep disorders), among others. [34,36,37,38,39]

Others

- *Pramipexole* is a dopamine agonist used to treat Parkinson's disease, which has no effect on pain but improves sleep quality in patients with fibromyalgia. [36,38,53,54]
- *Tizanidine* is a centrally acting alpha-agonist 2-adrenergic agonist that has an effect similar to muscle relaxants in patients with fibromyalgia. [36,38]

9. EFFECTIVENESS OF ANTIDEPRESSANTS AGENTS: A REVIEW

Based on a review of medical literature, using databases as PubMed, Cochrane, Lilacs and Medline, it was proposed as objective of this study the evaluation of antidepressant agents in the treatment of fibromyalgia, and subsequently in the depressive symptoms of the affected patients.

Table 6. Muscle relaxants used in FM treatment

Muscle Relaxants				
	Mechanism of Action	**Metabolism**	**Excre-tion**	**Common side effects**
Cycloben-zaprine [36,38,41,48]	Action center skeletal muscle relaxant, it reduces somatic motor activity by acting on alpha and gamma motor neurons.	Hepatic metabolism by CYP3A4, 1A2 and 2D6;	Urine and faeces	Dry mouth, drowsiness, dizziness

Table 7. Anxiolytics used in FM treatment

Anxiolytics				
	Mechanism of Action	**Metabolism**	**Excretion**	**Common side effects**
Alprazolam [36,38,40,41]	It binds to benzodiazepine receptors in the postsynaptic GABA neuron in the CNS. The inhibitory effect of GABA is due to increased neuronal membrane permeability to chloride ions, causing hyperpolarization.	Hepatic metabolism by CYP3A4	Urine	It increased or decreased appetite, sedation, constipation, weight gain or weight loss, fatigue, dry mouth, dysarthria, somnolence, memory impairment, depression, irritability
Clonazepam [36,45,46]	It depresses nerve transmission in the motor cortex suppressing the seizure discharge	Hepatic metabolism	Urine	Drowsiness is the most common
Zolpidem [36,47]	Selective affinity for alpha-1 of the omega-1 type GABA receptor. It increases GABAergic chloride conductance, hyperpolarizing neuronal membranes and reduces the excitatory activity.	Hepatic metabolism, mainly by CYP3A4	Urine, bile and faeces	Headache, drowsiness, dizziness
Zaleplon [36,38,40]	It interacts with the GABA receptor by binding to the benzodiazepine omega-1 receptor.	Metabolism mainly by aldehyde oxidize and a lesser extent by CYP3A4	Urine	Headache is the most common
Trazodone [36,38,40]	It inhibits the reuptake of serotonin, induces changes in presynaptic adrenoceptors of 5-HT, decreasing the sensitivity of this one. It also blocks histamine receptors (H1) and alpha1 adrenergic receptors.	Hepatic metabolism by CYP3A4	Urine and faeces	Nausea, sedation, headache, dry mouth, blurred vision, dizziness
Buspirone [36,38,40,41]	It has a high affinity for serotonin 5-HT1A and 5-HT2 receptors and moderate affinity for dopamine D2 receptors.	Hepatic metabolism by oxidation	Urine and faeces	Dizziness is the most common

Anxiolytics				
	Mechanism of Action	**Metabolism**	**Excretion**	**Common side effects**
Temazepam [36,38,40,41]	It binds to benzodiazepine receptors in the postsynaptic GABA neuron in the CNS. The inhibitory effect of GABA is due to increased neuronal membrane permeability to chloride ions, causing hyperpolarization.	Hepatic metabolism	Urine	Euphoria, Weakness, Confusion, Diarrhea, Hangover, Dizziness, Drowsiness, Lethargy, Vertigo
Sodium oxybate [36,38]	Derivative of GABA, it acts through specific receptors gamma-hydroxybutyrate (GHB) and GABA (B).	Metabolism via the Krebs cycle and beta-oxidation pathway	Pulmonary and urine	Headache, Nausea, Dizziness, Pain, Somnolence, Pharyngitis, Infection

Table 8. Anticonvulsivants used in FM treatment

Anticonvulsants				
	Mechanism of Action	**Metabolism**	**Excretion**	**Common side effects**
Pregabalin [36,37,38,50]	It binds to the alpha2-delta subunit of calcium channels inhibiting the release of excitatory neurotransmitter.	Metabolism insignificant	Urine	Ataxia, tremors, weight gain, somnolence, edema, dizziness
Gabapentin [36,38,49,50]	It binds to the alpha2-delta, structurally similar to pregabalin, but not approved for the treatment.	Metabolism insignificant	Urine	Dizziness, ataxia, drowsiness, fatigue, viral infection
Tiagabine [36,51,52]	Increases the activity of GABA by binding to its receptor. Inhibits the uptake in presynaptic neurons, increasing the availability of GABA.	Metabolism hepatic by CYP (mainly 3A4)	Faeces, urine and as unchanged drug	Nausea, weakness, tremors, dizziness, nervousness, reduced concentration, drowsiness

For this, it was selected only randomized controlled trials (RCT's), decreasing significantly the number of found studies.

In addition to antidepressant drugs, it was also found RCT's involving other drugs from other pharmacological classes, such as:

- Gabapentin [55]
- Naltrexone [56]
- Pramipexole [54]
- Pregabalin [57]
- Pyridostigmine [58]
- Sodium oxybate [59]
- Terguride [60]
- Dolasetron [61]

Altogether, 3 RCT's of antidepressant agents were found: (1) duloxetine, a selective inhibitor of serotonin reuptake, (2) milnacipran, a non-selective inhibitor of serotonin and noradrenalin reuptake, and finally (3) moclobemide, a monoamino oxidase inhibitor, and amitriptyline, a tricyclic antidepressant. [62,63,64]

The number of patients in each group (antidepressant x placebo-controlled) as well as primary and secondary outcomes were collected. The number needed to treat (NNT) or to harm (NNT), even as the size effect by Cohen's method.

9.1. Estimates

- NNT: 1/ARR, where ARR = lCER − EERl
* CER = control group event rate / EER = experimental group event rate

- Cohen's d:

$$d = \frac{\bar{x}_1 - \bar{x}_2}{s}, \qquad s = \sqrt{\frac{(n_1 - 1)s_1^2 + (n_2 - 1)s_2^2}{n_1 + n_2}},$$

(x = average / s: standard deviation)

$$s_1^2 = \frac{1}{n_1 - 1}\sum_{i=1}^{n_1}(x_{1,i} - \bar{x}_1)^2$$

Table 9. List of articles cited and discussed along the text

Paper	Journal / Year	Authors	Number of patients/ controls	Primary Outcome	Secondary Outcomes	NNT / NNH	Size Effect	Improvement of Depression
A double-blinded, multicenter trial comparing duloxetine with placebo in the treatment of fibromyalgia patients with or without major depressive disorder [62]	Arthritis & Reumatism 2004	Arnold LM *et al.*	104 X 103	Fibromyalgia Impact Questionnaire (FIQ) total score FIQ pain score	- Main tender point pain threshold - Number of tender points - FIQ fatigue - Tiredness on awakening - Stiffness scores - Clinical Global Impression of Severity Scale - Patient Global Impression of Improvement Scale - Brief Pain Inventory - Medical Outcomes Study Short Form 36 - Quality of Life in Depression Scale - Sheehan Disability Scale	NNT: 7,9; 95% Confidence Interval (4,2-76,6) Absolute Risk Reduction: 12,59%; 95% Confidence Interval (1,31-23,87%)	3,11 (analysis of impact in FIQ pain score) - 3,04 (analysis of Quality of Life in Depression Scale)	Although it was obtained a high value for Cohen's *d* (size effect) in scales involving depression, the study analyzed the effectiveness of duloxetine in several measures (as quoted in outcomes), and the results showed that this treatment is effective for most of them, in patients with or without fibromyalgia. Comments: An effective response involves a reduction of at least 50% in the FIQ pain score.

Table 9. (Continued)

Paper	Journal / Year	Authors	Number of patients/ controls	Primary Outcome	Secondary Outcomes	NNT / NNH	Size Effect	Improvement of Depression
Effectiveness and safety of milnacipran 100 mg/day in patients with fibromyalgia: results from a randomized, double-bind, placebo-controlled trial [63]	Arthritis & Reumatism 2010	Arnold LM *et al.*	516 X 509	Patient's Global Impression of Change (PGIC)	- Short Form 36 (SF-36) score - Pain Severity Score on Brief Pain Inventory - FIQ total score Multidimensional Fatigue Inventory	NNT: 6,3 ; 95% Confidence Interval (4,6-9,8) Absolute Risk Reduction: 15,93%; 95% Confidence Interval (10,22 − 21,64%	-5,87 (analysis of PGIC) 1,06 (analysis of mental component of SF-36)	The efficiency of milnacipran in depression was not evaluated based on appropriate scales for this psychiatric disorder. However, this drug proved to be effective in improvement of pain, fatigue, mental and physical functions.
A randomized, double-bind, placebo-controlled study of moclobemide and amitriptyline in the treatment of fibromyalgia in females without psychiatric disorder [64]	British Journal of Rheumatology 1998	Hannonen P *et al.*	43 (M) x 42 (A) x 45 (P)	Visual Analogue Scales (VAS)	Nottingham Health Profile Sheehan's Disability Scale	*Moclobemide:* NNT: 30,0 Confidence Interval (3,5 -) Absolut Risk Reduction: 3,33%; 95% Confidence Interval (- 21,96, +28,61) *Amitriptyline*	*Moclobemide* 0,15 (analysis of VAS) - 0,08 (Component "emotions" in NHS) *Amitriptyline* - 0,05 (analysis of	The study concluded that moclobemide must be not used in the treatment of FM. The researchers exclude the patients with depression, therefore, the role of these drugs in this psychiatric disorder cannot be evaluated. However, amitriptyline showed a moderate effect

Paper	Journal / Year	Authors	Number of patients/ controls	Primary Outcome	Secondary Outcomes	NNT / NNH	Size Effect	Improvement of Depression
						NNT: 4,0 Absolute Risk Reduction: 25% Confidence Interval (1,65-48,35%)	VAS) - 0,56 (Component "emotions" in NHS)	size when the emotional component was tackled. Comments The study involved a small number of participants in each group, with a high dropout rate in the complete follow-up.

CONCLUSION

This way, it becomes clear that fibromyalgia is still a challenge for the medical studies, since it covers countless associated symptoms and others comorbities.

Its pathophysiology remains obscure, being reported few advances in genetic researches, besides the absence of specific diagnostic exams. The clinical method, on the other hand, remains sovereign, the only one capable of determining its diagnosis.

As said before, the concomitance of psychiatric disturbances is very prevalent. And the depression, discussed on this chapter, is one of them. Here were showed the most recent treatments used in FM, like the antidepressant agents, and their mechanism of action and efficiency was established, through studies.

At the same time, very few of these studies have an A-1 level of evidence, characterized as randomized, double-bind, placebo-controlled clinical trials. And yet some of these some are based on their performance. And ultimately, some results, as shown by the estimates of NNT and size effect, were not favorable.

Therefore, it is noteworthy the need for the development of more RCT's involving antidepressant agents, since they are prescribed to patients with FM and have no proven efficiency.

REFERENCES

[1]   Clauw DW, Arnold LM, McCarberg BH *et al.* The science of fibromyalgia. *Mayo Clin Proc.* 2011 Sep;86(9):907-11.

[2]   Smith HS, Harris R, Claw D et al. Fibromyalgia: an afferent processing disorder leading to a complex pain generalized syndrome. *Pain Physician.* 2011 Mar-Apr;14(2):E217-45.

[3]   Köllner V, Bernard K, Bialas P *et al.* Diagnosis and therapy on fibromyalgia syndrome. *Psychother Psychosom Med Psychol.* 2011 Jun;61(6):276-85.

[4]   Arnold LM, Clauw DJ, McCaberg BH *et al.* Improving the recognition and diagnosis of fibromyalgia. *Mayo Clin Proc.* 2011 May;86(5):457-64.

[5]   Kassam A, Patten SB. Major depression, fibromyalgia and labour force participation: a population based cross-sectional study. *BMC Musculoskeletal Disorders* 2006, **7**:4.

[6]   History of Fibromyalgia. Available in < http://www.healthcentral. com/chronic-pain/fibromyalgia-287647-5.html> Accessed on December 3rd, 2011.

[7]   Hudson JI, Hudson MS, Pliner LF et al. Fibromyalgia and major affective disorder: A controlled phenomenology and family history study. *Am J Psychiatry* 1985; 142:441-446.

[8]   Marson P, Pasero G. Historical evolution of the concept of fibromyalgia: the main stages. *Reumatismo,* 2008; 60(4):301-304.

[9]   Spaeth M. Epidemiology, costs, and the economic burden of fibromyalgia. *Arthritis Research & Therapy* 2009, 11:117

[10]   Russell IJ, Raphael KG. Fibromyalgia Syndrome: Presentation, Diagnosis, Differential Diagnosis, and Vulnerability. *CNS Spectr. 2008;13:(3 Suppl 5):6-11.*

[11]   Shuster J, McCormack J, Pillai RR *et al.* Understanding the psychosocial profile of women with fibromyalgia syndrome. *Pain Res Manaq 2009,* May-Jun: 14(3):239-45.

[12]   Thieme K, Turk DC, Flor H. Comorbid depression and anxiety in fibromyalgia syndrome: relationship to somatic and psychosocial variables. *Psychosom Med 2004,* Nov-Dec: 66 (6):837-44.

[13]   Wolfe F, Ross K, Anderson J *et al.* The prevalence and characteristics of fibromyalgia in the general population. *Arthitis Rheum* 1995; 38:19-28.

[14]   Wolfe TA, Ross K, Anderson J, Russell J: Aspects of fibromyalgia in the general population: Sex, pain threshold, and Fibromyalgia symptoms. *J Rheumatol* 22: 151-6, 1995.

[15]   Wolfe F, Smythe HA, Yunus MB *et al.* The American College of Rheumatology 1990. Criteria for the classification of fibromyalgia. Report of the Multicenter Criteria Committee. *Arthritis and Rheumatism,* vol. 33, no. 2, pp. 160–172, 1990.

[16]   Wolfe F, Clauw DJ, Fitzchales MA *et al.* Fibromyalgia criteria and severity scales for clinical and epidemiological studies: a modification of the ACR preliminary diagnostic criteria for fibromyalgia. *Journal of Rheumatology,* vol. 38, no. 6, pp. 1113–1122, 2011.

[17]   Ceko M, Bushnell MC, Gracely RH. Neurobiology Underlying Fibromyalgia Symptoms. *Pain Research and Treatment,* vol. 2012.

[18] Yunus MB. Role of central sensitization in symptoms beyond muscle pain, and the evaluation of a patient with widespread pain. *Best Pract Res Clin Rheumatol.* 2007 Jun;21(3):481-97.

[19] Yunus MB. Fibromyalgia and overlapping disorders: the unifying concept of central sensitivity syndromes. *Semin Arthritis Rheum.* 2007 Jun;36(6):339-56.

[20] Arnold LM, Hudson JI, Keck PE *et al.* Comorbidity of fibromyalgia and psychiatric disorders. *J Clin Psychiatry.* 2006 Aug;67 (8):1219-25.

[21] Fietta P, Fietta P, Manganelli P. Fibromyalgia and psychiatric disorders. *Acta Biomed.* 2007 Aug;78(2):88-95.

[22] Abeles AM, Pillinger MH, Solitar BM *et al.* Narrative review: the pathophysiology of fibromyalgia. *Ann Intern Med.* 2007 May 15;146(10):726-34.

[23] Gracely RH, Petzke F, Wolf JM *et* al. Functional magnetic resonance imaging evidence of augmented pain processing in fibromyalgia. *Arthritis and Rheumatism,* vol. 46, no. 5, pp. 1333–1343, 2002.

[24] Lautenbacher S, Rollman GB, McCain GA. Multimethod assessment of experimental and clinical pain in patients with fibromyalgia. *Pain,* vol. 59, no. 1, pp. 45–53, 1994.

[25] Berglund B, Harju EL, Kosek E *et al.* Quantitative and qualitative perceptual analysis of cold dysesthesia and hyperalgesia in fibromyalgia. *Pain,* vol. 96, no. 1-2, pp. 177–187, 2002.

[26] Wood PB, Schweinhardt P, Jaeger E. Fibromyalgia patients show an abnormal dopamine response to pain, *European Journal of Neuroscience,* vol. 25, no. 12, pp. 3576–3582, 2007.

[27] Staud R, Vierck CJ, Cannon RL *et al.* Abnormal sensitization and temporal summation of second pain (wind-up) in patients with fibromyalgia syndrome. *Pain.* 2001;91:165-75.

[28] Boomershine CS. A Comprehensive Evaluation of Standardized Assessment Tools in the Diagnosis of Fibromyalgia and in the Assessment of Fibromyalgia Severity. *Pain Research and Treatment.* Volume 2012, Article ID 653714.

[29] Okifuji A *et al.* A standardized manual tender point survey. I. Development and determination of a threshold point for the identification of positive tender points in fibromyalgia syndrome. *J Rheumatol.* 1997 Feb; 24(2):377-83.

[30] Geisser et al. Perception of noxious and innocuous heat stimulation among healthy women and women with fibromyalgia: association with

mood, somatic focus, and catastrophizing. *Pain*, 102 (2003), pp. 243–250.

[31] Russell IJ, Larson AA. Neurophysiopathogenesis of fibromyalgia syndrome: a unified hypothesis. *Rheum Dis Clin North Am.* 2009 May;35(2):421-35.

[32] Martinez-Lavin M, Vargas A. Complex adaptive systems allostasis in fibromyalgia. *Rheum Dis Clin North Am.* 2009 May;35(2):285-98.

[33] Busch AJ et al. Exercise for treating fibromyalgia syndrome. *Cochrane Database Syst Rev*, 2007.

[34] Goldenberg DL. Multidisciplinary modalities in the treatment of fibromyalgia. *J Clin Psychiatry.* 2008;69 Suppl 2:30-4.

[35] Thieme K, Flor H, Turk DC. Psychological pain treatment in fibromyalgia syndrome: efficacy of operant behavioural and cognitive behavioural treatments. *Arthritis Res Ther.* 2006;8(4):R121.

[36] Winfield JB. Fibromyalgia Treatment. Available in < http://emedicine.medscape.com/article/329838> Accessed on December 09th, 2011.

[37] Häuser W, Bernardy K, Uçeyler N *et al.* Treatment of fibromyalgia syndrome with antidepressants: a meta-analysis. *JAMA.* Jan 14 2009;301(2):198-209.

[38] *Smith H, Bracken D, Smith J. Pharmacotherapy for Fibromyalgia. Pharmacol.* 2011; 2: 17.

[39] Häuser W et al. Treatment of fibromyalgia syndrome with antidepressants: a meta-analysis. *JAMA* 301:198, 2009.

[40] Smith B, Peterson K, Fu R *et al. Drug Class Review: Drugs for Fibromyalgia: Final Original Report.* Portland (OR): Oregon Health & Science University; 2011 Apr.

[41] Hauser W, Thieme K, Turk DC. Guidelines on the management of fibromyalgia syndrome - A systematic review. *Eur J Pain.* 2009.

[42] Montgomery SA. The place of milnacipran in clinical practice. *Int Clin Psychopharmacol.* 2003;18(Suppl 1):1–9.

[43] Dadabhoy D, Clauw DJ. Fibromyalgia - A Different Type of Pain. Therapy. *Nat Clin Pract Rheumatol.* 2006;2(7):364-372.

[44] Goldenberg DL, Burckhardt C, Crofford L. Management of fibromyalgia syndrome. *JAMA* 292:2388, 2004.

[45] Arnold LM. Strategies for managing fibromyalgia. *Am J Med* 122:S31, 2009.

[46] Mokhlesi B, Leikin JB, Murray P, et al. Adult Toxicology in Critical Care: Part II: Specific Poisonings. *Chest*, 2003, 123(3):897-922.

[47] Holm KJ, Goa KL. Zolpidem. An Update of Its Pharmacology, Therapeutic Efficacy and Tolerability in the Treatment of Insomnia. *Drugs*, 2000, 59(4):865-89.

[48] Winchell GA, King JD, Chavez-Eng CM, et al. Cyclobenzaprine Pharmacokinetics, Including the Effects of Age, Gender, and Hepatic Insufficiency. *J Clin Pharmacol*, 2002, 42(1):61-9.

[49] Brown JT, Randall A. Gabapentin Fails to Alter P/Q-Type Ca2+ Channel-Mediated Synaptic Transmission in the Hippocampus In Vitro. *Synapse*, 2005, 55(4):262-9.

[50] Sills GJ. The Mechanisms of Action of Gabapentin and Pregabalin. *Curr Opin Pharmacol*, 2006, 6(1):108-13.

[51] Adkins JC, Noble S. Tiagabine: A Review of Its Pharmacodynamic and Pharmacokinetic Properties and Therapeutic Potential in the Management of Epilepsy. *Drugs*, 1998, 55(3):437-60.

[52] Leach JP, Brodie MJ. Tiagabine. *Lancet*, 1998, 351(9097):203-7.

[53] Smith H, Bracken D, Smith J. Pharmacotherapy for Fibromyalgia. *Pharmacol.* 2011; 2: 17.

[54] Holman AJ, Myers RR. A randomized, double-blind, placebo-controlled trial of pramipexole, a dopamine agonist, in patients with fibromyalgia receiving concomitant medications. *Arthritis Rheum.* Aug 2005;52(8):2495-505.

[55] Arnold LM, Goldenberg DL, Stanford SB *et al. Gabapentin in the treatment of fibromyalgia: a randomized, double-bind, placebo-controlled, multicenter trial. Arthritis & Reumatism.* Vol. 56, No. 4, April 2007, pp 1336–1344.

[56] Younger JM, Zautra AJ, Cummins ET. *Effects of naltrexone on pain sensitivity and mood in fibromyalgia: no evidence for endogenous opioid pathophysiology.* Plos One. 2009, vol. 4.

[57] Crofford LJ, Rowbotham MC, Mease PJ *et al.* Pregabalin for the treatment of fibromyalgia syndrome. Results of a randomized, double-bind, placebo-controlled trial. *Arthritis & Reumatism.* Vol. 52, No. 4, April 2005, pp 1264-1273.

[58] Jones KD, Burckhardt CS, Deodhar AA *et al.* A six-month randomized controlled trial of exercise and pyridostigmine in the treatment of fibromyalgia. *Arthritis & Reumatism.* Vol. 58, No. 2, February 2008, pp 612-622.

[59] Russell IJ, Perkins AT, Michalek JE *et al.* Sodium oxybate relieves pain and improves function in fibromyalgia syndrome. *Arthritis & Reumatism.* Vol. 60, No. 1, January 2009, pp 299-309.

[60]   Distler O, Eich W, Dokoupilova E *et al*. Evaluation of the efficacy and
        safety of terguride in patients with fibromyalgia syndrome. Results of a
        twelve-week,   multicenter,   randomized,   double-blind,   placebo-
        controlled, parallel-group study. *Arthritis & Reumatism*. Vol. 62, No. 1,
        January 2010, pp 291-300.

[61]   Vergne-Salle P, Dufauret-Lombard C, Bonnet C *et al*. A randomized,
        double-blind   placebo-controlled   trial   of   dolasetron,   a   5-
        hydroxytryptamine 3 receptor antagonist, in patients with fibromyalgia.
        Eur J Pain. 2011 May;15(5):509-14.

[62]   Arnold LM, Lu Y, Crofford LJ *et al*. A double-bind, multicenter trial
        comparing duloxetine with placebo in the treatment of fibromyalgia
        patients with or without major depressive disorder. *Arthritis &
        Reumatism*. Vol. 50, No. 9, September 2004, pp 2974-2984.

[63]   Arnold LM, Gendreau RM, Palmer RH *et al*. Efficacy and safety of
        milnacipran 100 mg/day in patients with fibromyalgia: results of a
        randomized,   double-blind,   placebo-controlled   trial.   *Arthritis &
        Reumatism*. Vol. 62, No. 9, September 2010, pp 2745-2756.

INDEX

G

H

I

Q

R

worldwide, 52

X

xerostomia, 45, 47

Y

yield, 50